"If there is another book that does a better job of demonstrating how the polyvagal theory is applied to group treatment interventions with teenagers and adults, I am unaware of its existence. This essential and thought-provoking work provides the reader with all of the strategies needed to apply the polyvagal approach to life. It is chock full of experiential exercises that are empirically based and executed with clinical perspicacity. The co-authors Montano and Iadeluca are to be commended for producing a novel work, which will be an asset to anyone who embraces it. I highly recommend this book to anyone interested in utilizing this approach."

Frank M. Dattilio, *PhD ABPP, Clinical Professor of Psychiatry, University of Pennsylvania Perlman School of Medicine and teaching associate (part time), Harvard Medical School*

"In *Polyvagal Theory in Group Practice*, Antonella Montano and Valentina Iadeluca skillfully translate Stephen Porges' and Deb Dana's insights into a transformative journey for groups. This heartfelt and reader-friendly book empowers mental health professionals, educators, and community leaders to apply the '*Wired to Connect*' program, fostering impactful change across various contexts. Emphasizing experiential learning, readers will not only grasp the theory but also integrate its principles into their daily practice and real-world experiences. The book is enriched with beautifully created images that enhance understanding, motivation, and engagement. It is a 'must-read' source for anyone interested in promoting resilience and connection within diverse groups without leaving anyone or any groups behind. Thank you both for this precious book you have written!"

Mehmet Zihni Sungur, *Professor of Psychiatry, Istanbul Kent University, Istanbul; President of the Turkish Association for Cognitive Behavioural Therapies (TACBT); Founding Fellow, Certified Supervisor, Diplomate, Trainer, Consultant Academy of Cognitive Therapy (ACT); Beck Institute International Advisory Committee*

I0084497

Polyvagal Theory in Group Practice

This book describes *Wired to Connect*, a 10-week program for groups based on Polyvagal Theory that is structured, easy to teach, and suitable for everyone. The course is designed to help people develop an awareness of how their autonomic nervous system affects them as they navigate the joys and challenges of life, and how to embrace and modulate its reactions to lead a more serene and fulfilling existence.

It begins with an introduction to the theory and functioning of the autonomic nervous system, whose biological response to safety and danger – real or perceived – can determine whether a person is in a state of open connectedness or mobilized/immobilized protectiveness. It continues by reviewing the knowledge and skills required to lead the program, along with an overview of its structure and the various teaching modules that, like building blocks, form each class.

The second part of the book serves as a manual for leading the course. Going session by session, activity by activity, it offers specific, hands-on scripts to help convey the theory to course participants in a simple and engaging way, along with experiential exercises on breath, movement, and sounds, as well as homework assignments and guided immersions into mindfulness. Valuable teaching aids – such as color plates, audio tracks, and slides – are available for download to assist the instructor in guiding their students through the *Wired to Connect* journey.

Not only can psychologists and psychotherapists lead the program, but also other compassionate professionals, such as teachers, doctors, nurses, and community workers. *Polyvagal Theory in Group Practice* is a clear, concise, and comprehensive handbook for anyone interested in learning how to benefit from a polyvagal lifestyle and to share this knowledge with others.

Antonella Montano is a CBT psychotherapist and Founder and Director of the A.T. Beck Institute for Cognitive Behavioral Therapy in Rome and Caserta. She is a Certified Trainer/Consultant/Supervisor of A-CBT (Academy of Cognitive and Behavioral Therapies) and Member of the Beck Institute International Advisory Committee. She teaches CBT and mindfulness-based protocols, and she is a public speaker and author of numerous publications, including more than 20 books, book chapters, and scientific articles.

Valentina Iadeluca is a psychologist, somatic psychotherapist, and certified Hakomi teacher, with advanced training in mindfulness-based therapeutic modalities and CBT. She is the author of several psychology books and Executive Co-Director of the Hakomi Institute of Mallorca, the English-language European headquarters of Hakomi Mindful Somatic Psychotherapy. She is engaged at the forefront of teaching Hakomi throughout Europe. She complements her formal education with nearly 20 years of continuous personal growth through meditation and yoga practices. In her previous career, Valentina was a professional singer and music educator.

Polyvagal Theory in Group Practice

Wired to Connect

Antonella Montano and Valentina Iadeluca
Translated by Anna C. Forster

Routledge
Taylor & Francis Group

LONDON AND NEW YORK

Designed cover image: The Polyvagal House © Istituto A.T. Beck, Sophie
Ajello

First published in English 2026

by Routledge
4 Park Square, Milton Park, Abingdon, Oxon OX14 4RN

and by Routledge
605 Third Avenue, New York, NY 10158

Routledge is an imprint of the Taylor & Francis Group, an informa business

© 2026 Antonella Montano and Valentina Iadeluca

Published in Italian by Edizioni Centro Studi Erickson 2023
La Teoria Polivagale in Pratica
© 2023 by Edizioni Centro Studi Erickson, Trento (Italy)
All rights reserved.
www.erickson.it
www.erickson.international

Translated by Anna C. Forster

Published in Italian by Edizioni Centro Studi Erickson 2023

British Library Cataloguing-in-Publication Data
A catalogue record for this book is available from the British Library

ISBN: 978-1-032-91023-9 (hbk)
ISBN: 978-1-032-91018-5 (pbk)
ISBN: 978-1-003-56096-8 (ebk)

DOI: 10.4324/9781003560968

Typeset in Times New Roman
by Deanta Global Publishing Services, Chennai, India

Access the Support Material: www.routledge.com/9781032910185

Contents

PART II

Program Description

Session 1 Our Autonomic Nervous System: A Story That Began Long Ago 31

Session 2 The Key Principles of Polyvagal Theory

Session 3 Lights, Shadows, and Bridges

Foreword

This book is about the complexity and wonders of a part of our body called the autonomic nervous system (ANS). Generally speaking, we know little about it, and we certainly do not take it much into account when reflecting on our health. If I think back to my medical training (in the early 1990s), I notice an obvious disconnect; from anatomy to physiology, I was taught a lot of complex information, but this did not find much application in practice. The general idea was to learn the basic functions of the body. While these things were obviously important for us to know, it would be up to researchers and neurophysiologists to study them in depth. We clinicians, instead, would be tasked with recognizing and distinguishing between individual diseases (differential diagnosis), understanding how they work inside the body (pathophysiology), and treating people directly. The only exception was perhaps clinical management of cardiac arrhythmias, however "niche" the topic may have seemed to us students, busy learning a little bit of everything.

At that time, however, came a neurophysiologist, Stephen Porges, who would change everything. He was studying a particular type of arrhythmia and came up with a model that greatly expanded the scope of our understanding of the ANS. In doing so, he created an important bridge between physiology and practice. Porges was researching a very delicate clinical field: extremely premature babies. This was the 1970s, when great strides were being made in neonatology. The survival and protection of children from the most frequent causes of serious diseases (mostly metabolic and infectious) was vastly improving. Nonetheless, and despite having overcome many of these frailties, some of these children sadly died. The cause was found to be so-called "arrhythmic storms", when their hearts beat so fast that they could no longer stand the strain.

Unlike the "standard" arrhythmias that can occur at any age of life, the problem was not the heart and its electrical regulatory network. In full-term infants, the action of the ANS to restore normal heart rate is taken for granted. In preterm infants, however, this basic function has not yet fully developed. The issue was, therefore, both complex and tragic. This intuition prompted Stephen Porges to "take the path of the vagus nerve". Since then, he has been our leading light. He has provided us clinicians with one insight after another and broadened our view on the importance of the ANS for individual and relational health. His talent was, and still is, his ability to distinguish previously ignored facets and complexities in vagal functioning.

Prior to his observations, the classical theory was binary and rather simplistic. It considered ANS function as like a set of scales. On one side was the parasympathetic/vagal system, the "calming" side (and the oldest in evolutionary terms), which was balanced by the other side, the "exciting" (ortho)sympathetic/adrenergic system (more recently evolved). If the question of saving pre-term infants was as simple as balancing the scales, it would be enough to pharmacologically or electrically stimulate the vagal system. This remedy was obviously attempted and was, at least in part, effective. However, as Porges wrote, recalling an Anglo-Saxon motto, "even too much of a good thing is a bad thing". Indeed, the problem was not only the heart beating too fast (tachycardia), but also too slowly (bradycardia). In such children the vagus nerve was overactive, and stimulating it would be counterproductive. In fact, when this was attempted, the scales shifted from one extreme to another, in a sort of double storm, before they died. There was, therefore, some key piece of information missing, one that Porges would intuitively unlock. Surprisingly, some of these ANS crises quieted when the newborn was held. It might seem obvious to us nowadays, when the so-called kangaroo mother care (prolonged contact between a pre-term infant and one of the parents) is routine, but at that time it was a revolutionary idea. Indeed, until then, neonatologists had been almost exclusively preoccupied by preventing fatal infections, and premature babies were isolated to ensure maximum sterility.

Touch is an important part of our relations with other people: even when we meet someone new, the first thing we do is shake hands. The same is true for premature infants. They might know practically nothing of the world, but they do grasp the benefits of touch: they are instinctively calmed and comforted by physical contact. They perceive this and embody it through their ANS.

Since it is calming, the mechanism must have a vagal foundation. However, at the same time it seems to be operating at a higher level than the "basic" cholinergic activity of the parasympathetic nervous system, responsible for ensuring healthy heart rate and activation of the anabolic rest and digestion, energy absorption, and waste evacuation systems. Indeed, in these newborns, Porges began to notice and measure a specific type of vagal activity that "senses" the relationship with the other. In other words, it understands that the infant is safe. As such, it can switch off both orthosympathetic and parasympathetic alarm systems, since they are not needed at that time.

Thus it emerged that we have two different vagal "modes", which naturally needed different names. Porges defined the oldest and more basic mode the "dorsal vagal" and the more recent and complex the "ventral vagal". The model he proposed would therefore be termed polyvagal. The formation of this theoretical framework has had profound and far-reaching practical consequences. Before it, the concern was to protect pre-term infants by shielding them from infections. Now, their need for tactile contact, to activate a deep sense of security, is understood. This "higher" vagal activity was operating above both the sympathetic system and the "lower" vagal system.

The second practical consequence of Porges' theory was the finding that, as in other serious diseases, an insufficient response to treatment is often due to focusing on the patient's problem, without paying sufficient attention or working to enhance their existing resources. The lesson learned from the treatment of arrhythmias in pre-term babies, as well as many other diseases that benefit from the approach, was that polyvagal resources are ancestral, deep-rooted, and powerful. They make us profoundly resilient mammals. As the title of this book says, they are "wired" into our ANS, its hierarchy, and its many potential tasks.

The ANS immediately works to assess a threat (neuroception) and respond to it appropriately (fight, flight, or freeze). Where no danger has been detected, instead, the ventral vagal system allows threat-free proximity and connectedness, creating the ideal ground for higher cognitive and relational functions such as care, coopera- tion, and social play, as well as metacognitive and self-reflective states.

Drawing inspiration from the ideas of mental health professionals like Deb Dana, the book you are about to read is also a valuable resource. It presents a program for groups, framing these ideas in a clear and concise manner. The result is a ten-session journey on which participants are encouraged to listen to and befriend their own ANS, exercising it consciously and gently. They are taught how to integrate these exercises into their daily routine and thereby live a calmer, more reflective life. The characteristics and qualities of the ideal polyvagal instruc- tor are also outlined. Indeed, it is the professional and personal experience of the authors, Antonella Montano and Valentina Iadeluca, that give this book added value. Their skills range from cognitive-behavioral therapy to somatic approaches such as Hakomi, yoga, voice work, and ethnomusicology. Their insights and exper- tise shine through, enriching the book and making it deeply convincing. Happy reading!

Giovanni Tagliavini, Psychiatrist, Psychotherapist,
President of the Italian Association for the
Study of Trauma and Dissociation (AISTED)

Preface

Like everything we have done together, *Wired to Connect* was inspired by our life experiences – what intrigues and fascinates us personally. It grew out of our shared openness to new challenges, our love of learning, and our desire to look beyond the confines of what is known and familiar to us.

For both of us, the creation of this protocol represented a new opportunity for insight into the field of psychotherapy. This voyage of discovery led us down two paths. On the one hand, we enhanced our knowledge of neurophysiology, in a top-down approach, while on the other, we immersed ourselves in practical activities, following a bottom-up trajectory. We attended courses with Stephen Porges himself – the father of Polyvagal Theory – as well as with Deb Dana and Arielle Schwartz, who translated that theory into operational tools. With our respective backgrounds, we delved into various disciplines, such as meditative practices, yoga, singing and music, and different kinds of somatic techniques. We looked at this multiplicity of experiences through a polyvagal lens. Exploring our personal responses enabled us to verify their very impact on our autonomic nervous system and savor the benefits in terms of our own regulation.

The next step was to pass this set of resources on to our patients, collecting their feedback as we went. This book represents the culmination of this process. It is designed to show you how we organized our knowledge and experience into *Wired to Connect*, a polyvagal program for groups. Through it, we aim to share Polyvagal Theory and its practical applications with as many people as possible. We have already tried and tested the protocol several times. The results achieved have been extremely encouraging in terms of both reducing symptoms of depression and anxiety and increasing emotional regulation skills.

The book will guide you on a similar journey and equip you with all the tools necessary to lead the program. The first chapter in Part I is dedicated to the theory behind what we like to call the *polyvagal revolution*. This compels us to rethink not only the general architecture of the autonomic nervous system, but also how human beings construct sense and meaning from their biological foundations. Care professionals will be encouraged to redefine their ways of conceptualizing suffering. The various activities presented here will provide them with a multimodal toolkit for treating discomfort in its somatic, emotional, and cognitive dimensions.

The second chapter focuses on the figure of the polyvagal instructor. It illustrates their ideal personal qualities, the set of tools they use, and the knowledge they need to acquire in order to lead the *Wired to Connect* program. This information is simplified and condensed into a particular section, a sort of teachers' handbook that can be readily consulted at any time.

The third chapter offers a detailed overview of the program, outlining the structure, target audience, working methodology, and logistical aspects. It explains the rationale behind the different learning modules that, like building blocks, compose every class.

Part II describes the program session by session, activity by activity. It includes specific scripts to help future instructors explain the theory to course participants and convey even complex content in the most engaging way. Of course, while leading the protocol, we encourage you to adapt our suggestions to your own personal style.

The experiential exercises that focus on breathing, sound, and movement represent a distinctive feature of *Wired to Connect*. We have attempted to describe every single step of them as meticulously as possible and make them accessible to everyone. The same is true for the homework assignments and the guided imageries, both pillars of the protocol.

The volume contains illustrations that we specifically created to accompany the program. They clarify key aspects and enrich the experience of the participants. The online resources that complement the book can be downloaded via the URL found at the bottom of page vi. These include PowerPoint presentation models for each session, which you can use as a guide for creating your own. All plates are also available in color, and are useful for introducing the Polyvagal Theory to clients and generating your own slides. Further downloadable resources are the texts for the guided imageries, pictures of the yoga asanas, and the audio tracks (mantras, songs, sound inputs) used during Session 7, which is dedicated to sound.

It is now time to delve into the book and, most of all, try *Wired to Connect* for yourself. A gentle reminder: the ability to communicate with your own nervous system is built primarily upon experience. We hope that, once you have finished reading, you will want to roll up your sleeves and embrace the spirit behind this program with an open mind and heart. Whatever your discipline, polyvagal awareness should help you enrich the lives of your participants, helping them understand the role played by their physiology in their overall well-being. Armed with this knowledge, they should be better equipped to face challenges and lead their existence from a somatic space of safety and regulation.

Antonella Montano and Valentina Iadeluca

Wired to Connect

What Is It and How Does It Work?

Chapter 1

Before We Begin

1.1 Our Stories Begin in the Body: Why a Group Program on Polyvagal Theory?

What enables some people to respond to day-to-day challenges effectively and creatively? Where do they get the agility and resilience to handle unpleasant events, problems, pain, and frustration?

The answer is: the flexibility of their nervous system.

Think about it: the way we experience life, love, and failure, and our ability to get back on our feet when we fall, depends on how our bodies have learned to respond to certain stimuli over time and how quickly we can adjust. Generally speaking, this happens without us being aware of it – a kind of knee-jerk reaction. In other words, the stories we tell ourselves about both who we are and what the world is like begin in our body. Our feelings – fear, anxiety, sadness, serenity, and joy – originate in our organs, our guts, our muscles, and our joints.

Now we can use a different lens to view how our mind and body interact: a construct called Polyvagal Theory. This new way of understanding the human nervous system was developed by American neuroscientist and psychiatrist Stephen Porges (1995, 1998, 2001, 2007, 2009, 2021; Porges & Dana, 2018) in the mid-1990s. It postulates that the vagus nerve – the tenth cranial nerve – which connects the brain to the intestine, plays a vital role in our response to safety or danger signals from our environment. As their primary processor, it switches on our autonomic nervous system (ANS). This prepares our body for connection, or alternatively for fight, flight, or freeze; it decides for us whether we will mobilize or immobilize when faced with a threat.

These behavioral responses have evolved over hundreds of thousands of years. They dictate how we react to age-old questions such as: *Is that a predator I hear approaching? Have I got time to run, or should I play dead to save myself? Can I trust you to help me? Can I trust myself?* They also lay the organic foundations of our feelings, underpinning our emotional, cognitive, and somatic spheres.

As human beings, we all, without exception, share this evolutionary conditioning. When we feel safe, we are calm, open, and engaged; when we feel threatened, we can either mobilize to defend ourselves or beat a retreat or, alternatively, play

DOI: 10.4324/9781003560968-2

possum to shield ourselves from harm. Only when we feel completely safe can we connect to ourselves, to others, and to the reality that surrounds us, not to mention the divine or the supernatural. Only then do we have the energy to effectively face the difficulties of life and to fully savor its joys.

Thus, safety and interpersonal relationships are the biological imperatives that underlie the complex architecture of our ANS. Polyvagal Theory sheds light on these, explaining how they unfold in sequence, and the close connections between them. It also suggests a pathway for us to work on to modulate our automatic ANS-mediated responses and to stop leading our existence in fight, flight, or freeze mode.

But how can we react to things that happen faster than we can consciously perceive them? How can we "tune out" the constant barrage of danger signals in our daily lives – the stress of home, family, work, war, climate change, etc.? Many of us are haunted by a constant perception of alarm and feelings of not being able to cope. What do we do when we are overwhelmed and just want to throw in the towel and take refuge within ourselves?

Well, the good news is that Polyvagal Theory is not just a theory. The construct has been translated into a series of operational tools, thanks to Stephen Porges' cooperation with other mental health specialists. In particular, Deb Dana (2018, 2020, 2021), an expert complex trauma therapist and Coordinator of the Traumatic Stress Research Consortium at the Kinsey Institute in the United States, has been instrumental in turning Porges' theory into therapeutic practice. She has developed a series of techniques to help people live more consciously in their bodies and build an alliance with their nervous systems. The goal is to achieve a better equilibrium and thus be able to take greater control of their lives.

As Dana says (2021, p. 2):

When the inner workings of our biology are a mystery, we feel as if we are at the mercy of unknown, unexplainable and unpredictable experiences. Once we know how our nervous system works, we can work with it. As we learn the art of befriending our nervous system, we learn to become active operators of this essential system.

It is to Deb Dana and Stephen Porges that we extend our heartfelt thanks: without them, neither our program nor this book would exist today. We are convinced that the widespread application in society of the theoretical and practical resources inspired by their work can promote personal and collective well-being. It can help alleviate discomfort and suffering in the face of fear, aggression, isolation, and relational poverty. This is the reason why we have devised *Wired to Connect*. The program organizes polyvagal knowledge and skills into a structured voyage of self-discovery and experiential learning for groups. Suitable for schools, group homes, therapy groups, prisons, hospitals, and many other settings, the ultimate goal is to foster polyvagal awareness within small and large communities.

As such, *Wired to Connect* guides its participants, directing their attention towards their own ANS and helping them understand how it works. Once they have learned to speak its language, they will be empowered to use it to write a new narrative for their own lives.

The participants begin their journey by familiarizing themselves with how the ANS – an extraordinary apparatus – is organized and activated. They continue by getting to know the succession of connection, mobilization, and immobilization states that generate our experiences moment by moment. This process is not only mental. It is *embodied*, involving profound feeling and sensing from within, with every fiber of our being. Building on this awareness, specific exercises can be practiced to re-educate the nervous system, teaching it to react flexibly to the demands of everyday life, whether ordinary or unexpected. The goal is to find a safe space inside, especially as we face what challenges lie ahead. We should all dwell in this baseline state for as long as possible and learn to return to it when pulled away. Specific neural patterns are activated when we perceive that we are secure and protected. Switching on these synaptic connections voluntarily and repeatedly is essential: after all, practice makes perfect. Once we experience how our ANS operates, we can learn to regulate it, making us better prepared for the future. This understanding progressively paves the way to a different way of inhabiting our skin. The destination is a place in which it is possible to enjoy solitude, bask in beauty, and derive nourishment from the gaze of others without the need for barriers of any kind.

1.2 Who Is This Book For?

The volume is primarily intended for psychologists, psychotherapists, teachers, educators, community workers, and physiotherapists who are interested in becoming instructors and offering the program to groups of teenagers or adults. However, it is important to note that reading this book is only a starting point: before you can teach the various activities suggested, you will need to try them directly and practice them until they become an integral part of your day. Acquiring a polyvagal approach to life means learning to communicate with your own nervous system. You can only arrive at the cognitive through the somatic; you must experience it in the first person and truly make it your own before you can share your knowledge and skills with others.

We therefore encourage you to spend time testing the program on yourself. Once you incorporate a polyvagal perspective into your day-to-day life, you will begin to reap the rewards. In doing so, you will develop a skill set and basic attitude that will allow you to fully grasp not only the many nuances of your own autonomic world, but also those experienced by the members of the group you are instructing. In other words, once you have mastered the art of polyvagal exploration and modulation, you will be able to tune in to the responses of your participants' nervous systems and gently guide them towards connection and regulation.

Chapter 2

The Polyvagal Instructor
Everything You Need to Know to Run the Program Well

Who can conduct *Wired to Connect*? What knowledge and skills should they possess? This chapter attempts to answer these questions comprehensively. The first section focuses on the polyvagal instructor's personal characteristics and distinctive leadership style. The second outlines the basics of Polyvagal Theory that are essential for teaching the program. Finally, the third section explores the operational tools that the instructor should master in order to lead the various exercises effectively. The combination of these elements will allow the teacher to handle *Wired to Connect* with ease and to make it an exciting and transformative experience for program participants.

2.1 The Polyvagal Instructor

It is not only mental health specialists who can lead *Wired to Connect*. Anyone who feels they have the appropriate experience, vocation, and interest in group management can try their hand at teaching it. However, whatever your professional background, it is important that as a polyvagal instructor you operate within the professional boundaries established by law in your country. Also, we cannot stress enough the importance of the instructor's role in ensuring that the program reaches and renews the hearts of participants.

Before you start, you must have a good grounding in Polyvagal Theory and have personally experienced the content offered to the group to be able to convey it with authority and credibility. You must have experimented with the exercises yourself. You will thus be an expert in your own autonomic universe and know how to read the activation states of the members of the group you lead. In short, you will have developed a *polyvagal approach to life*.

In addition, there is no learning without safety. And this is all the more true when you are working to shed light on the autonomic responses of participants to certain stimuli. Indeed, these can be associated with feelings of shame and interpreted as signs of inadequacy. We encourage you, as a polyvagal instructor, to interact with the group from a state of genuine interest and honest acceptance. This means being curious about other people's experiences, inviting them to embark on a journey of self-discovery of their own autonomic nervous system (ANS), and

DOI: 10.4324/9781003560968-3

celebrating their innate intelligence at every opportunity. We suggest providing information on the rationale behind the various exercises, – the why, the what, and the how – whenever possible. The nervous system needs to understand in order to feel safe and trust.

In a process that involves autonomic responses, non-verbal language is as important as words, if not more so. Remember that how you move and express yourself, using your voice and gaze, can inspire confidence and calm. The atmosphere you create should engage the group and encourage their active cooperation. Keep your attention open, welcoming, and attuned. Your role is to maintain a state of regulation and model this energy. That means fostering authentic relationships, identifying moments of disengagement, and guiding participants back to connection. The ability to illuminate the sequence of polyvagal states is key. Make room for emotions and embrace them firmly. Use your nervous system in service of the group's learning process.

Think of a tablespoon of salt in a glass of water. The mixture will be very salty, practically impossible to drink. But if you pour that same mixture into a larger container, a pool of water or a lake, the salt will be less evident, if at all. As a polyvagal instructor you are that lake. You contain and dilute an enormous amount of emotional material. You allow sadness and pain to coexist alongside joy and happiness. If positive feelings enter the room, point them out and encourage participants to savor them whenever possible.

2.2 Polyvagal Theory at a Glance

Here we provide an overview of the principles that underlie Polyvagal Theory, as illustrated by Porges (1995, 1998, 2001, 2007, 2018, 2021) and Dana (2018, 2020, 2021) in their various publications. It is possible – and advisable – to reinforce and expand upon the information provided in this book by reading the original sources. We strongly encourage you, as a novice polyvagal instructor, to review this set of knowledge before you address it in session with a group.

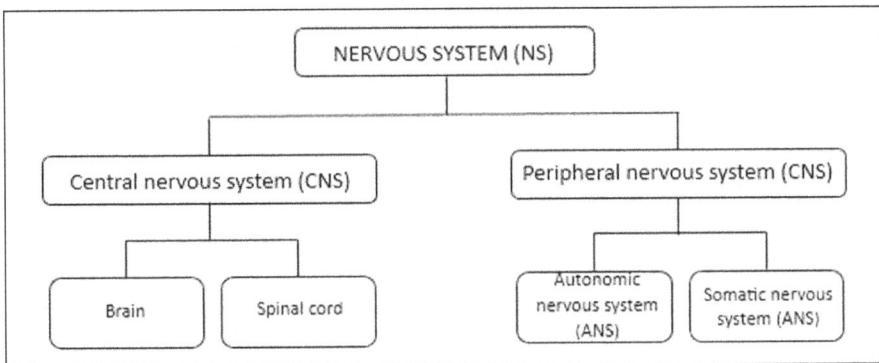

Figure 0.1 The Central and Peripheral Nervous Systems.

2.2.1 The Polyvagal Basics: The ABCs of the Human Nervous System

As shown in Figure 0.1, the human nervous system has two basic parts: central and peripheral. The central nervous system (CNS) is made up of the brain and spinal cord. It controls most of the body's voluntary functions, including consciousness, movement, thought, speech, and our five senses (sight, hearing, smell, taste, and touch). The peripheral nervous system (PNS), on the other hand, is composed of the set of nerves and ganglia outside the brain and spinal cord. Its main function is to maintain a link between the CNS and the rest of the body.

In turn, the PNS is divided into the somatic nervous system (SNS) and the autonomic nervous system. The SNS is associated with voluntary control of movements through the action of skeletal muscles. The ANS, on the other hand, acts largely involuntarily and regulates bodily functions such as heart rate, breathing, pupillary responses, bladder, and sexual responses. The ANS is the shining star of *Wired to Connect*. Let us see why.

2.2.2 The Origins of Polyvagal Theory

Polyvagal Theory was developed by the American psychiatrist Stephen W. Porges and presented for the first time to the scientific community in Atlanta at the Congress of the Society for Psychological Research on 8 October 1994. It takes its name from the vagus nerve (Figure 0.2), the tenth cranial nerve; *poly* comes from the Greek adjective *polys*, which means *many*. This prefix reminds us that the nerve is made up of a family of different pathways. "Vagal" comes from the Latin *vagare*, i.e., wandering. Indeed, it follows a long and intricate path inside the human body, starting its journey at the base of the head, then passing through the chest and descending to the depths of the bowels.

It has two branches, leading it in two directions. From the diaphragm upwards it connects to the heart, lungs, pharynx, and larynx. This tract of the nerve is called the *ventral vagal*. Here its fibers are myelinated, meaning that information travels through them extremely quickly and efficiently. The ventral vagal influences the heart and respiratory rates and integrates with the facial nerves, forming the "social engagement system" (see Section 2.2.5 dedicated to this topic). From the diaphragm down, on the other hand, the nerve connects the stomach, liver, spleen, kidneys, and intestines. This section, mainly unmyelinated, is defined as the *dorsal vagal*, which affects the organs responsible for digestion and sexual response.

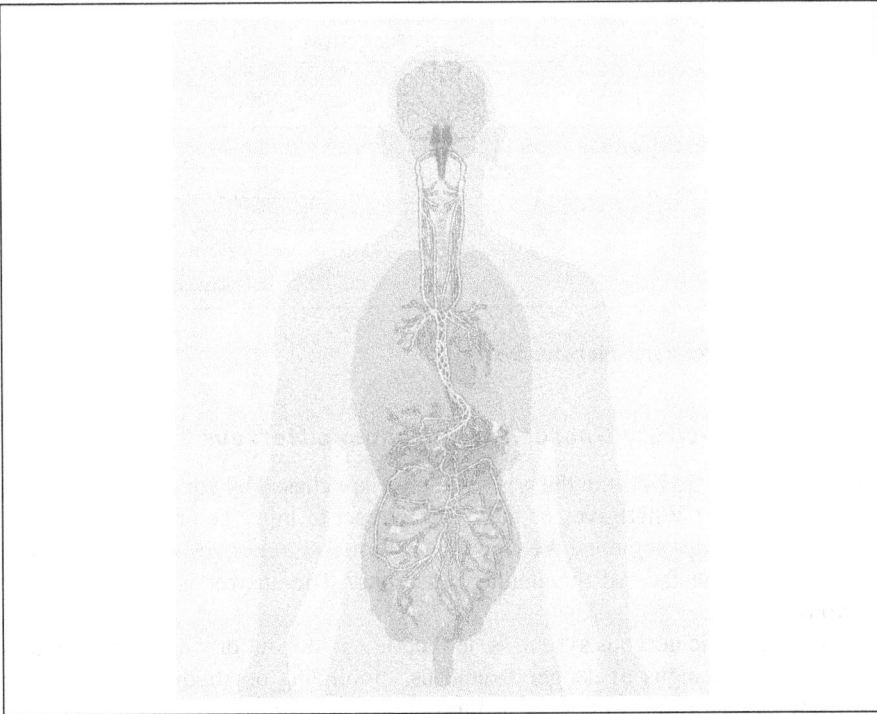

Figure 0.2 The Vagus Nerve.
Copyright: Axel Kock, used with permission.

Why did we say that the autonomic nervous system is the star of *Wired to Connect*? Because Polyvagal Theory – as illustrated in the diagram that follows (Figure 0.3) – redraws its map, going beyond the traditional division into sympathetic and parasympathetic and proposing a new structure, or rather a new hierarchy of response:

- Ventral vagal pathway.
- Sympathetic pathway.
- Dorsal vagal pathway.

Through these three pathways, "we react in service of survival" (Dana, 2018, p. 22). This vocabulary can be complex at first. But in these words, there lies a real revolution: they represent the language of safety and human connection.

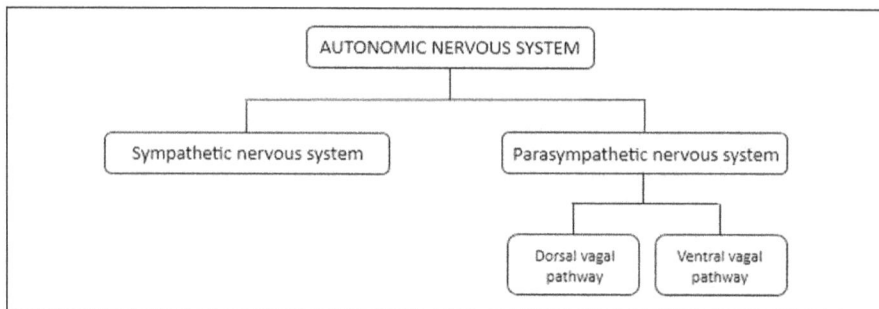

Figure 0.3 The Autonomic Nervous System.

2.2.3   *Our Security Guard: The Autonomic Nervous System*

How are we able to run like the wind when we are chased by someone we believe wants to hurt us? What gives us the drive to react to injustice or violence perpetrated against us or someone we care about? Which force saves our lives, immobilizing us in the face of threatening situations? The answer is: our autonomic nervous system.

The autonomic nervous system is, in fact, like a lookout or watchman. It reacts to even the first signs of danger around us, mobilizing our body to perform the most appropriate action at that particular moment, even before our conscious mind understands what is happening.

We can all agree that an immediate physiological response – preparing us to fight, flee, or freeze – enables us to do just what it takes to survive when confronted with violence, assault, robbery, natural disaster, etc. However, there are other situations that can lead to a "false alarm", causing us to overreact: for example, taking a crowded subway, preparing for an important business appointment, having a medical exam, arriving at a party where we don't know anyone, or being asked a question in class. While we are in no real danger, we may sense a threat that our body reacts to in the same way it would to a risk to life.

Why, then, does our autonomic nervous system process certain cues, and not others, as *dangerous* or *safe*? And why do we tend to overreact in certain situations as if they were threatening, while they are objectively not?

The way in which our individual nervous system automatically interprets certain stimuli and responds to them is forged by the set of experiences we shared with our caregivers in the very first years of our lives. What we felt inside the womb, the welcoming gaze at the moment we were born, the type of contact we received in the very first days of our existence, the atmosphere we lived in at home during childhood, the educational style of our main attachment figures, any episodes of mistreatment, abuse, or bullying, and so on. All this takes root within us, shaping how our nervous system reacts to certain stimuli and, consequently, how we respond through a cluster of bodily, emotional, and cognitive processes. This explains why some people are essentially at peace with themselves, whereas others are inhabited by prevailing feelings of alarm or experience a sense of exclusion from the game of life. Finally, there are still others who constantly shift between restlessness and alienation. Somehow, their stories began in the past. Yet, it is never too late to regain a sense of control over things that once seemed beyond us and to build a cozier and more reassuring autonomic home for ourselves.

2.2.4   The Basic Principles of Polyvagal Theory

Polyvagal Theory is built around three founding principles: *autonomic hierarchy*, *neuroception*, and *co-regulation*. Let us analyze them one by one.

2.2.4.1   The Autonomic Hierarchy

Just like the brain, the autonomic nervous system has developed over time, with its three sections – dorsal vagal, sympathetic, and ventral vagal (Figure 0.4) – progressively building on each other. These three systems are activated in response to cues of safety and danger, which trigger specific behavioral patterns through a certain set of physical sensations, urges, impulses to action, emotions, and thoughts.

The dorsal vagal section is the oldest. It dates back to about 500 million years ago and is common to all vertebrates. It uses immobilization ("playing possum") as an extreme defense response, the last bastion in the face of stimuli perceived as highly threatening to our safety. When the dorsal vagal autonomic state is activated, we tend to *freeze*: we feel numb, frozen, drained, absent, collapsed, dissociated: essentially "scared to death" (Figure 0.5).

The next section to develop was the sympathetic system, about 400 million years ago. It enables us to react in the face of possible danger through mobilization. It triggers responses of *fight or flight*: we either approach/attack or seek distance/escape. In this state, people feel agitated, apprehensive, anxious, worried. Being sociable and forming connections are a distant concern (Figure 0.5).

The ventral vagal system appeared last, about 200 million years ago. Mammals have one, but reptiles do not. It mediates responses of connection and social engagement. It makes relationships, intimacy, and play possible, based on an autonomic foundation of trust and security (Figure 0.5).

The activation of these states is governed by a precise hierarchy, that is to say, it follows a specific sequence. From the ventral vagal state, the detection of objective or subjective danger makes us move towards sympathetic mobilization. From here, when the threat persists or we do not feel able to face it, we move towards dorsal vagal shutdown/collapse. There is only one way to move out of these states: from dorsal vagal immobilization we need to pass through sympathetic mobilization to return to ventral vagal connection.

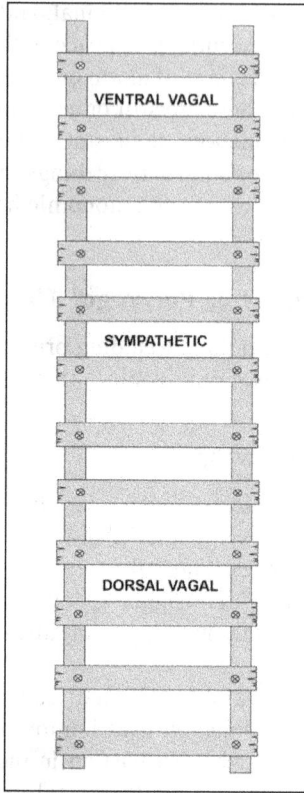

Figure 0.4 The Autonomic Hierarchy.

From *The Polyvagal Theory in Therapy: Engaging the Rhythm of Regulation* by Deb Dana. Copyright © 2018 by Deb Dana. Used by permission of W. W. Norton & Company, Inc.

As Dana herself proposed (2018, p. 10), this hierarchical organization of our autonomic universe can be represented graphically through the image of a ladder (Figure 0.4 and Figure 0.6). On the highest rungs is the ventral vagal state, in the center the sympathetic, and at the bottom the dorsal vagal. When we are in the ventral vagal state, the common obstacles of everyday life do not seem so alarming to us. When we get a flat tire, leave our phone at home, or are late for work, instead of getting angry or anxious, we are able to accept it and go along with the flow. If, however, many small difficulties begin to build up on one another, or when we experience a single event that our nervous system interprets as overwhelming, we tumble down the ladder. We no longer feel safe, and we are unable to maintain a calm view of reality. Instead, we react by attacking or fleeing. If we then continue to feel trapped in an endless cycle of problems with no apparent way out, we

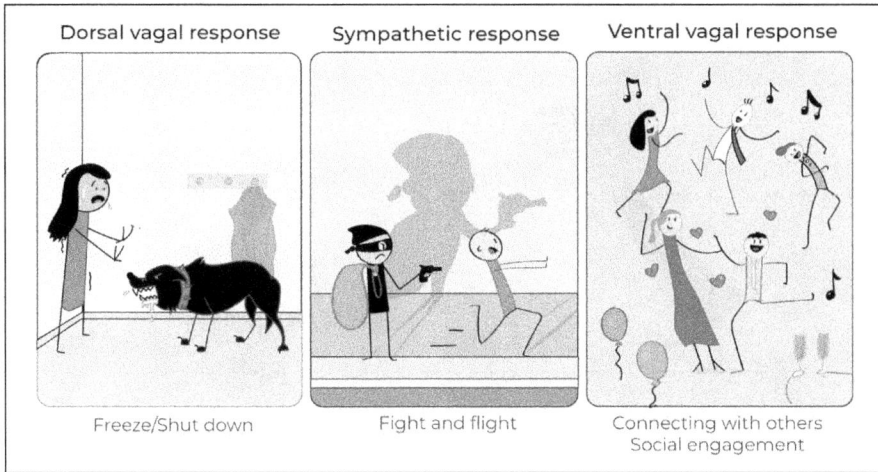

Dorsal vagal response   Sympathetic response   Ventral vagal response

Freeze/Shut down   Fight and flight   Connecting with others Social engagement

Figure 0.5 The Evolution of the Nervous System and Its Three Stages of Response.

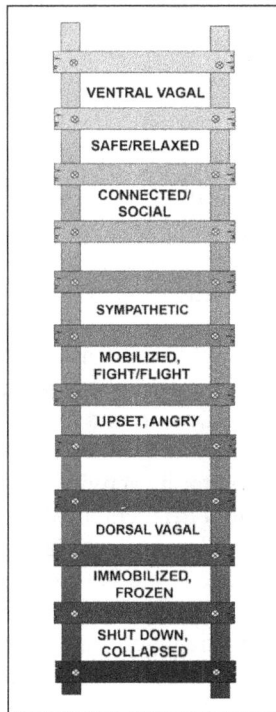

VENTRAL VAGAL

SAFE/RELAXED

CONNECTED/ SOCIAL

SYMPATHETIC

MOBILIZED, FIGHT/FLIGHT

UPSET, ANGRY

DORSAL VAGAL

IMMOBILIZED, FROZEN

SHUT DOWN, COLLAPSED

Figure 0.6 The Autonomic States and Their Characteristics.

From *The Polyvagal Theory in Therapy: Engaging the Rhythm of Regulation* by Deb Dana. Copyright © 2018 by Deb Dana. Used by permission of W. W. Norton & Company, Inc.

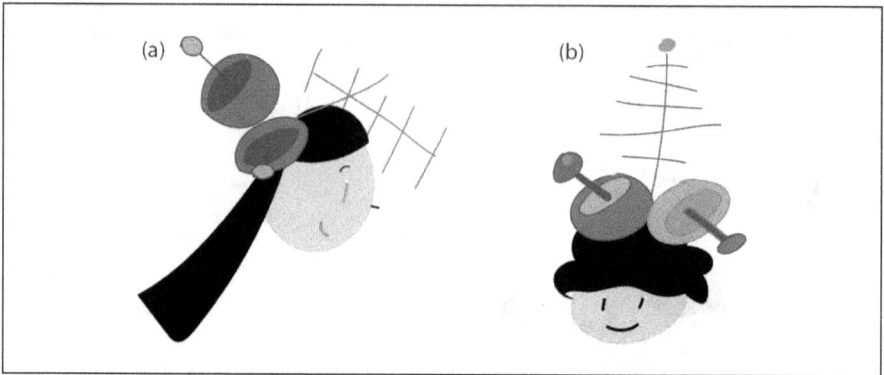

Figure 0.7 (a) and (b) Neuroception.

plummet even further down: we slip into dorsal vagal activation and therefore feel frozen, shut down, closed off.

It should be noted that between one state and another, there are several intermediate states, each with various nuances. In the course of our day, we move from the activation of one system to another. Fortunately, most of the time, we do not spend too long in distressing sympathetic mobilization or dorsal vagal shutdown.

2.2.4.2 Neuroception

Polyvagal Theory explains that we all possess a sort of surveillance system, almost like a sense that acts below our thinking brain. This is called neuroception. We can imagine neuroception as a set of antennas or sensors (Figure 0.7). These sensors are present in our body and are constantly working to understand:

- our internal environment: our physical sensations, emotions and thoughts;
- our external environment: what is happening around us;
- our interpersonal space: the others around us.

The purpose of this incessant monitoring activity is to detect cues of safety (which Dana calls "glimmers") or danger ("triggers"). When a danger signal is detected, it initiates changes in our body to prepare us to face the potential threat. Through neuroception we pass from one autonomic state to another.

Normally, we are not aware of the stimuli that result in the transition from ventral vagal serenity to sympathetic mobilization, and from there down to dorsal vagal immobilization, but we are perfectly aware of the bodily responses that follow. In other words, our biology changes long before the information reaches our conscious mind.

As previously mentioned, our personal life experiences dictate whether our neuroception interprets a signal as threatening or safe. If our autonomic nervous system was formed in a dysfunctional environment, this can lead to "neuroceptive incongruence", a faulty threat-assessment system: either we are unable to remain calm in objectively safe contexts or we cannot activate an adequate defense in high-risk conditions. In other words, our habitual autonomic responses tend to be over- or under-reactive, keeping us trapped in the narrow confines of a distorted reality built for us many years ago.

2.2.4.3 Co-regulation

The third principle at the foundation of Polyvagal Theory establishes that we are "wired to connect", that is, our nervous system is designed for connection with others (Figure 0.8). When we are safe and serene, we can interact well with the people around us, who in turn help us remain emotionally stable. This dynamic process is called "co-regulation", an innate need that accompanies us from the beginning of our lives and never leaves us. We come into the world unable to provide for ourselves, and are therefore totally dependent on our caregivers. We rely on the adults around us to meet our needs, which are not only physical but also emotional and psychological. As well as the air we breathe and the milk we need to grow and become capable of taking care of ourselves independently, we need reassurance, love, and human contact. If all has gone well enough during our development, as adults we will move quite effortlessly between moments of connection with ourselves, our surroundings, and the people who give meaning and significance to our existence.

Our need to mutually co-regulate persists throughout the course of our life. It is an essential component of our well-being, but it is also a challenge. Indeed, the biological imperative of connection walks hand in hand with our other primary

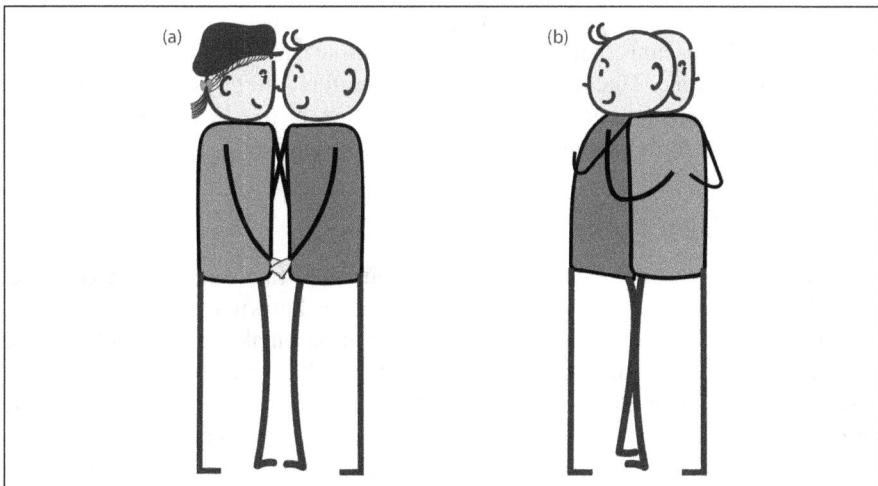

Figure 0.8 (a) and (b) Co-regulation.

need: safety. Only when we feel safe can we open up, love, and trust others. Only then can we let our mind-body systems work in sync. Co-regulation is a subtle game that involves the gaze, voice, heart rate, breath, and all our affectivity, our ability to experience feelings and emotions. When such seeds of connection fall onto soil that our neuroception cannot trust to nurture them, the autonomic nervous system goes into defensive mode. We are driven to protect ourselves and we do so by attacking, fleeing, shielding ourselves, or shutting down.

Our society is built on the myth that we are independent beings, capable of self-regulation. Despite the pervasive messages to the contrary, at the foundation of our human nature is co-regulation. We need bonds, healthy bonds, arms to which we can return, friendly eyes to send us signals of solidarity, empathy, and security when the going gets tough out there. Our most important co-regulators are other people.

2.2.5   The Social Engagement System

The Social Engagement System is another fundamental construct of Polyvagal Theory. It is composed of the network of nerve pathways arising from the connections between the ventral vagus and the nerves that control our facial expressions, speech, and hearing: the fifth (trigeminal), seventh (facial), ninth (glossopharyngeal), and eleventh (accessory) cranial nerves. As Dana says, through the Social Engagement System, the human species is endowed with "a real organic connection between heart and face" (2021, p. 41).

The construct of the Social Engagement System is closely linked to the principle of co-regulation. Its activity translates into a set of body signals through which one person's nervous system sends messages of openness or closed-offness to the other. Based on cues from head movements, facial expressions, gaze, and voice, the Social Engagement System forms an assessment well before we are aware of whether or not we feel safe and comfortable with the person we are interacting with. Before a conscious thought is formed, we *know* whether we are welcome and able to trust someone. Thanks to this process, therefore, our physiology prepares to co-regulate through another or, instead, to fight, flee, or freeze, i.e., to unleash our innate autonomic mobilization or immobilization responses.

2.2.6   The Vagal Brake

A section of the ventral vagus nerve governs our heart rate, keeping it constant at around 72 beats per minute. This regulating action is known as the "vagal brake". By connecting to the sinoatrial node – our natural pacemaker – this ventral vagal component controls the amount of energy arriving at the heart from the sympathetic system, moment by moment. Think of the brakes on a bicycle: when you apply the brake the bike slows down, and when you loosen your grip, you can speed up. In the same way, the incoming energy rapidly decreases and the heartbeat slows down when the vagal brake is applied. When it is loosened, more energy is transferred and, consequently, the heart beats faster. In short, the vagal brake acts to adjust our heart rate so that we go about our daily lives without uncontrolled descent into the fight/flight sympathetic response. We can use the vagal break to move flexibly from states of defense and mobilization into states of regulation. From this perspective, the concept of the vagal brake can be linked to that of *resilience*, our ability to regain our equilibrium after a negative experience. It can be seen as an anchor, a lifeline that allows us to rise safely back to the calm surface of ventral vagal energy after being plunged into the tormented waters of sympathetic activation.

All of this is essential for the polyvagal instructor to understand. The exercises proposed by the program are also designed to help participants experiment with a series of intervention strategies to raise awareness of their vagal brake and learn tools to exercise control over it. This way, they can consciously climb their autonomous ladder and open up, as fully as possible, to the experience of safety and connection.

2.2.7   The Autonomic Impact of Trauma

There are many types of trauma that we might experience during our life. However, for the purposes of this book, we can broadly divide them into two categories. There are traumas arising from clearly recognizable individual episodes, such as earthquakes, car accidents, robberies, murder, etc., that are characterized by the experience of a sense of threat to life. There are also developmental traumas which occur during our childhood in the places where and at the hands of the persons with whom we should feel safe. These may be either harmful actions (verbal or non-verbal violence, abuse, etc.) or shortcomings (neglect, abandonment, inconstant care, etc.) that are protracted over time and can compromise our physical and emotional well-being.

We have seen how children are dependent on the adults who co-regulate them. We have also emphasized that safety and connection are two biological imperatives. Growing up within highly dysfunctional environments, in which our relationships with adults around us are unreliable and/or harmful, therefore, has a strong impact on the reactivity of our autonomic nervous system. In such situations, the child does not learn the skills that are necessary to co-regulate and is completely reliant on self-regulation. Having our biological needs unmet in such a fashion leads to feelings of loneliness and profound distress. As a result, our habitual autonomic responses tend to crystallize near the bottom of the ladder. Some individuals, therefore, end up living in fight-or-flight mode due to the ongoing activation of the sympathetic nervous system. Others, on the other hand, live life in standby, shut off from the world in a constant state of dorsal vagal immobilization. Both have only rarely, or even never, experienced the joy and peace of ventral vagal energy.

While these reactions serve a protective function, they prevent connection and make the world seem a very bleak or scary place. Living life stuck between the narrow confines of mainly survival responses is a source of great suffering. Hence, the instructor must be able to convey the fact that *change is possible*. Trauma survivors can learn to recognize their moments of dysregulation and, therefore, to expand and move more flexibly within their autonomic landscape. The encouraging polyvagal message is that we all possess the resources we need to bask in warm and reassuring ventral vagal energy. All we need to do is to learn how to unlock them.

2.2.8   Mixed States

Mixed vagal states allow mobilization and immobilization to be experienced from a place of ventral vagal connection and safety. As such, they re-educate the nervous system to dwell in the area of regulation. They progressively reduce the spectrum of neuroception triggers capable of activating the danger and survival responses of fight/flight or shutdown/collapse.

2.2.8.1   Ventral Vagal + Sympathetic

When the activating energy of the sympathetic meets the soothing calm of the ventral vagal, we enter "play mode", a specific autonomic state in which it is possible to dance, play, and open up with joy to other people. In other words, this is a great state to be in. Our vagal brake is working to our advantage, helping us to move with rapidity and ease between relaxation and action.

2.2.8.2   Ventral Vagal + Dorsal Vagal

Immobility puts a strain on our autonomic nervous system. It is difficult to stay still without switching off. However, there are circumstances in which the dorsal vagal and ventral vagal systems can cooperate to give the experience of immobility itself the flavor of safety, without experiencing dissociation. Examples of these are some forms of meditation, Yoga, Qi Gong, or deep relaxation exercises. Furthermore, it is natural for us to be still and motionless, as we experience the powerful force of connection in moments of intimate sharing with friends, a partner, or our children. We also enter this state when we cross the threshold between wakefulness and sleep, letting ourselves fall into the arms of Morpheus, warmed by the physical presence of someone who loves us.

2.3   The Polyvagal Instructor's Toolkit

Let us now analyze the practical skills that the polyvagal instructor must acquire in order to easily teach the various learning modules of the program, which will be described in detail in the next chapter. Here is a brief list:

- Present theoretical contents clearly and simply, using captivating and stimulating language that speaks to people's hearts.
- Lead experiential activities by modeling them in person while accompanying the participants through all the various steps.
- Guide the construction of the various polyvagal maps (Dana, 2018, p. 55) – the Personal Profile map, the Map of Lights and Shadows, the Regulating

Resources map – in class and/or assigned as homework. You must know them inside and out and have a profound understanding of their value. As Dana (2018, p. 54) says, these tools are "practical representations of [a participant's] autonomic nervous system at work". Over time, maps that were once confined to paper evolve into a sort of internal compass. Through this, people learn to recognize both their state of autonomic activation, the things that led them to where they are, and the set of personal and relational resources at their disposal to aid them in bringing themselves back into a regulated state.

Chapter 3

Program Organization

3.1 General Structure

Wired to Connect involves a minimum of nine meetings, one a week, each lasting about 2.5–3 hours. The program culminates in an 8-hour class – the *Safety and Connection Day* – to consolidate and reinforce what participants have learned.

As it unfolds, the program targets four main learning objectives:

- Understanding the functioning of the autonomic nervous system (ANS) at both cognitive and experiential levels.
- Recognizing the different autonomic states and their triggers.
- Acquiring tools to emerge from fight/flight (mobilization) and shutdown/collapse (immobilization) responses. This also means spending as much time as possible in a baseline "safe space", which allows people to connect to themselves, others, and the world around them.
- Consolidating and integrating this new knowledge and skills into everyday life.

Wired to Connect is like a tower, in which each learning module builds on the previous one. Hence, every session begins by reviewing the content and activities of the last class through a shared discussion of the assigned homework. The only exception is Session 1, which starts with participants introducing themselves to each other, and then diving into the first module's theory and experiential activities. Due to this stepwise organization, full attendance is desirable.

3.2 Participants: Who Can Benefit?

Wired to Connect is a program for everyone. Each of us has a nervous system. We all migrate between states of connection, mobilization, immobilization, and the many nuances in between. Understanding the effects of these biological processes on our lives and working on them can be an enlightening and transformative process for anyone.

By applying Polyvagal Theory and its tools, program participants learn to access and regulate their internal and interpersonal worlds. In essence, these tools

DOI: 10.4324/9781003560968-4

are emotional, bodily, cognitive, and behavioral techniques that enable effective intervention in almost everyone's autonomic landscape.

At its inception, Porges' work helped us better understand the neurophysiology of trauma. It advanced our knowledge of the reasons why the autonomic responses of people who suffered such wounds stiffen into attack or shutdown patterns. It shed light on how trauma can compromise the ability to flexibly return to a state of emotional and behavioral regulation (Levine, 1997; 2010; 2015; Van Der Kolk, 1996; 2003; Ogden & Fisher, 2015; Fisher, 2019). Hence, participation in *Wired to Connect* can certainly benefit those affected by post-traumatic stress disorder. However, it is important to note that, in such cases, the group instructor must be a mental health professional with specific training in trauma.

In addition, by further clarifying the relationship between mind and body from a neuroscientific perspective, Polyvagal Theory has recently paved the way for integrated operational models to treat a wide range of other psychological disorders (Porges and Dana, 2018). Therefore, the program is also suitable for specific clinical populations such as patients suffering from anxiety or mood disorders. In this case too, the instructor should be a trained psychologist or psychotherapist.

In short, only people experiencing an acute psychotic episode should be discouraged from participating in the program. That being said, in the interests of good practice, we advise assessing the suitability of each potential *Wired to Connect* participant via a thorough preliminary interview and, if possible, appropriate testing. We recommend the Beck Depression Inventory (BDI-II), the Hamilton Anxiety Rating Scale (HAM-A), the Symptom Checklist (Scl90), and the Difficulties in Emotion Regulation Scale (DERS) for this purpose.

3.3 How Does It Work?

As outlined in the descriptions of the various learning modules that make up the sessions, *Wired to Connect* is designed to involve multiple dimensions of a person's experience: cognitive understanding, feeling from within, experimenting, and meta-reflecting. Therefore, the approach is *multimodal*.

Each theoretical component is accompanied by experiential activities. In this program, *understanding by doing* is key. The course aims for participants to develop a refined perception of their own body and, thus, the ability to interact with their own nervous system. Engaging in practical exercises is the only way to achieve this goal.

As you work through the sessions, you will realize that we deliberately chose to offer different stimuli in each class. The aim is to be as inclusive as possible, reaching and inspiring people with very different backgrounds and learning styles.

3.4 A Typical Session

The program features a series of learning modules that fit together like building blocks. The order of the learning modules presented in this book is not, however, set in stone. With experience you will learn how to adjust the program to ensure that the class's learning goals are met as effectively as possible.

Below is a list of the five stages in a typical session. A detailed description of each is presented on the following pages.

1   Session opening and homework review
2   Polyvagal Theory Module
3   Experiential activities and sharing of personal experiences
4   Explanation and assignment of homework
5   Closing ritual

Now, let us analyze the various stages in more detail.

3.4.1   Session Opening

Each session starts with a welcome to the group. This is followed by a brief review of the theory and contents of the previous session, which aims to build a bridge to the main topic of the current class.

3.4.2   Homework Review

The homework set is always based on the theory and activities covered in class. It allows participants to continue developing their knowledge and skills on multiple levels – cognitive, emotional, and bodily – between sessions. As such, it represents a fundamental step in their learning process, giving them the opportunity to integrate Polyvagal Theory into their daily lives. We advise dedicating time to highlighting the importance of homework and encouraging the group to engage actively with it.

To promote adherence, we suggest that you ask participants to send their completed worksheets, video clips, etc., back (to you or your administrative assistant) via e-mail no later than four days after class. That way, you will have time to read them thoroughly, prepare for the next session, and follow up on any late submissions.

We recommend creating a slide presentation (e.g., PowerPoint) of participants' homework to be shared with the group as a whole. However, you must be sure to align with confidentiality laws in your country and your own sensibilities. If appropriate, you must present this option to the participants during the first session and ensure that everyone agrees. To this end, it is advisable to get each group member to sign an informed consent form. If a person feels uncomfortable with this level of disclosure, the point is not to force them. Instead, consider their needs or wishes and explore their reluctance in a private conversation.

As for the homework tasks themselves, there are two types: worksheet-based and experiential.

3.4.2.1   Worksheet-Based Homework

Although always rooted in participants' bodily awareness, written assignments aim to promote cognitive understanding of their autonomic world. We have already discussed the importance of constructing the various maps proposed in the first part of the program. Charting allows us to assign words and structure to the silent tangle of our biological responses, and to grasp their impact on our physical experience. It helps us give voice to the kind of thoughts about ourselves, others, and the world that we tend to produce when we are in a certain autonomic state. It enables us to sharpen our focus on the set of personal, relational, and environmental resources we possess that can help us re-emerge from a state of mobilization/immobilization.

In addition to making the various maps, the group is guided through self-exploration activities to gather information about the context in which their individual ANS was forged. This process culminates in a specific homework worksheet designed to give them deeper insight into the relationship between their past experiences and present reactions.

3.4.2.2 Experiential Tasks

These involve reproducing the activities learned in sessions at home. Repetition familiarizes participants with the various skills they absorb in class. Hence, they must always be encouraged to practice them and study their effects on their autonomic responses as often as possible. The idea is for each member of the group to develop a repertoire of experiences that allows them to consciously switch on the neuronal patterns associated with safety and connection, and to master modulating their states of activation.

Sharing and commenting on homework is a vital component of *Wired to Connect*. Therefore, giving ample time and attention during the session to this learning activity is crucial. This section of the session should last 60 minutes at most, during which, ideally, all homework submissions should be read and discussed together.

Below, we provide three options for best conducting the homework sharing and review. As an instructor, you should select the most appropriate one based on the size and sensibilities of the group and the number of leaders in attendance.

- *Model 1* (recommended for small groups): each participant reads their homework while the others listen without commenting. Then, the instructor – attentive, solicitous, and involved – can initiate the discussion. You should take care not only to foster the person's understanding but also to perform your function as a nervous system co-regulator. The group as a whole can learn from this exchange while actively training their attunement "muscles" and practicing empathetic listening and compassion.
- *Model 2* (recommended for large groups with two leaders): the group is divided into two subgroups, each led by an instructor, who conducts the homework review as indicated in Model 1.
- *Model 3* (recommended for large groups with one instructor): the group is divided into several subgroups of three people. Each subgroup, working in parallel, has about 30 minutes for its participants to read their homework, one at a time, and discuss it with their classmates. Then, the subgroups gather

together, and the instructor initiates a group discussion on the topics that emerged during the first part. Alternatively, you may focus on sharing and reviewing a selection of the worksheets received (remember, however, to carefully examine *all* participants' homework before the session).

3.4.3   Polyvagal Theory Modules

In each session, the instructor outlines the fundamental concepts of a particular aspect of Polyvagal Theory, as described in Chapter 2, introducing it step by step as the course unfolds. You can find a session-by-session overview of the program and the main topics related to it at the end of this chapter (Table 3.1). The class begins with a review of the principles covered in the previous meeting.

Offering theoretical content as engagingly as possible is crucial to the program's success. Explanatory images and graphics can be highly beneficial to this end. A series of illustrations and handouts that can be shared with the group are provided with this book. They can also be downloaded in color from the website using the URL found at the bottom of page vi. Visual aids promote understanding of the concepts presented, bringing them to life and consequently aiding learning. For the same reason, the theory modules dramatically benefit from the support of slide presentations (e.g., PowerPoint), or printed handouts in situations where projection is not possible. Presentation templates for each session are also available in the online resources. You can use them as a starting point in developing your own material.

Although transmission of this type of content necessarily involves an instructor-led teaching style, we encourage you to keep up a lively exchange with the group. We suggest actively involving the participants through the use of questions that stimulate them to develop personal reflections on the topics covered.

3.4.4   Experiential Activities

Experiential learning is one of *Wired to Connect*'s most essential and distinctive features. As stated in Chapter 1, Polyvagal Theory helps us understand that our stories begin in our body. Hence, the practical component is key to the program's success.

We have seen how our nervous system reacts to certain stimuli, prompting our physiology to respond to them. These modifications play a major role in how we feel overall. In other words, there is a direct link between our autonomic nervous system's responses and the cluster of physical sensations, motor impulses, emotions, and thoughts that determine our behavior.

The good news is that the reverse is also true: our behavior, i.e., the actions we perform each day, whether large or small, can modulate the habitual responses of our autonomic nervous system. This means it can be re-educated, allowing us to dwell in that baseline safe space from which connection is possible. This is why this type of learning is so critical: it allows people to directly experience the beneficial power of polyvagal activities and exercises, inspiring them to add this toolkit of resources to their everyday lives.

The course involves two types of experiential activities: guided imagery and breathing, sound, and movement exercises.

3.4.4.1 Guided Imagery

The aim of guided imagery activities is to immerse participants in the visceral experience of their own autonomic states. They are a kind of led self-exploration that triggers connection, mobilization, or immobilization responses just enough to study and embrace them without being overwhelmed. This process allows participants to develop an embodied understanding of their reactions, which they can use as a point of reference to monitor the succession of ventral vagal–sympathetic–dorsal vagal activation cycles – and the many nuances in between – we all experience during the day. Practicing the simple visualization of situations in which we feel calm, protected, at one with nature, or warmed by someone's presence can also evoke similar sensations in the here and now. They trigger the same neuronal patterns of connection and security, promoting the remodeling of autonomic responses and directing them towards regulation.

The guided imagery activities are also a way of cultivating the mindful stance of an empathetic observer. Through them, participants can learn to view the vagaries of their autonomic reactions through a benevolent and compassionate gaze.

3.4.4.2 Breathwork, Sound, and Movement Exercises

These draw inspiration from the bottom-up techniques typical of working with trauma, as well as age-old yoga and meditation practices, singing, and music. All these disciplines have intuitively interpreted our need for regulation and connection, which are integral parts of human nature and biology. For this reason, we have always meditated, sung, danced, and played, fully expressing our joyful feeling of being alive as we do so. Through these activities – simple, achievable, and practicable almost anywhere – the group experiences a set of actions designed to stimulate the vagus nerve and widen their window of emotional tolerance. The variety of techniques presented allows each participant to choose the ones that work best for their own autonomic nervous system.

3.4.5 Sharing of Personal Experiences

At the end of every activity in the program, we advise dedicating time for participants to share their feelings and thoughts. The instructor can prompt this by asking questions such as:

- How did your nervous system respond when…?
- What state was your ANS in when you started? What feelings, sensations, or thoughts told you that you were there?

- What autonomic state did you enter after…? And what feelings, sensations, or thoughts told you that you had arrived there?
- What did you observe in your body when…?
- What kind of emotions did you experience when…?
- What kind of thoughts did you tend to have when…?

This exchange allows the instructor to interpret the group's experience from a polyvagal perspective and provide feedback, thereby enhancing learning. In a safe, welcoming, and non-judgmental environment, the participants begin to open up and experience, in real time, the power of connection with both the instructor and the other members of the group.

3.4.6 Setting Homework

We encourage you to dedicate a specific part of the session to assigning home-work, ensuring that the whole group understands the instructions. You can choose whether to provide supplementary material, e.g., the slides used during class or audio/video recordings, to guide practice of the experiential activities at home. In this case, it is advisable to check that the whole group is able to easily access such resources and to take all necessary steps to resolve any technical/logistical difficulties they might experience.

3.4.7 Closing Ritual

Each session is concluded via a specific activity that, depending on the case, focuses on breathing, movement, or both. In this way, the session ends with the group practicing a tool for modulating the nervous system, ensuring that they return to their daily lives in a condition of awareness and regulation.

3.5 The Logistics

3.5.1 Group Size

The course can be delivered to a minimum of 6–8 people up to a maximum of 20–22. Bear in mind, though, that some people feel threatened by large groups. Hence, the larger the number of participants, the greater the care that must be taken to create a safe space. As we have seen, a sense of security is essential for working to understand and regulate autonomic states.

3.5.2 The Teaching Team

If the group is large, having both a lead instructor and a co-instructor may be help-ful. The latter can help to keep a close eye on what each participant is experiencing. They can also aid the instructor in managing the group and leading any activities carried out in small groups. The co-instructor may also take over specific exercises to enable the lead instructor to modulate their own autonomic state if needed. This should allow you to reopen to interaction with the group from a basis of co-regulating serenity.

We also advise recruiting an administrative aide to support the program by collecting homework and maintaining contact with the participants week to week.

3.5.3 Delivery

There is no doubt that bodily, emotional, and cognitive work focusing on the responses of the autonomic nervous system is best delivered in person. Being part of a physical group allows participants to explore their own reactions to the interpersonal experiences that the course provides. If all goes well, such interaction will enable individuals to connect with themselves, their fellow travelers, and their instructor, and experience the benefits of co-regulation in real time.

That said, it can be difficult for some people to attend a program consistently over the course of about three months. Hence, there is the option of online delivery. We have tested this approach, and although it is not ideal, it is certainly viable. It is essential, however, to stimulate people to give online meetings the same attention they would when attending in person. All must be fully present, fully there, even when learning at a distance. They should participate actively in all discussions and activities and keep the webcam on from the beginning to end of sessions. Under these conditions, participants can still learn a great deal about themselves and, as if by magic, the biological imperative of relationship manages to break through the barrier of the screen. At a certain point, people begin to feel like part of a group. If you choose the option of conducting the program online, we advise offering the last meeting – the *Safety and Connection Day* – as an in-person class.

3.5.4 Equipment

Whether you conduct the program in person or online, we suggest creating a messaging group (e.g., WhatsApp) and/or mailing list to exchange information on scheduling and homework between sessions.

The necessary equipment depends on the format you choose. For the face-to-face setting you will need:

- A spacious environment, proportionate to the group, with chairs, meditation mats, and cushions.
- A video projector and projection screen or, alternatively, printed handouts to be given to every participant at the beginning of each session.
- A whiteboard or a flipchart.
- Paper, markers, and colored pencils.

On the other hand, for the online setting a video conferencing platform (e.g., Zoom) is indispensable. Participants must provide the materials necessary to carry out the various activities (mats, colored pencils, etc.).

In either case, every group member should also have their own:

- Folder for keeping handouts, homework worksheets, and any other paper materials.

3.6 Overview of Sessions

Table 3.1 A Session-by-session Overview of the *Wired to Connect* Program

Session	Module
Session 1	Our Autonomic Nervous System: A Story that Began Long Ago
Session 2	The Key Principles of Polyvagal Theory
Session 3	Lights, Shadows, and Bridges
Session 4	Personal Resources
Session 5	The Vagal Brake
Session 6	Breathwork
Session 7	Sound
Session 8	Movement
Session 9	A Polyvagal Approach to Life
Session 10	Safety and Connection Day

Part II

Program Description

Our Autonomic Nervous System

A Story That Began Long Ago

The primary goal of the first session is to establish a polyvagal work environment within the group. This foundation will enable participants to open up to the experience of safety and connection with you and their fellow travelers. From the program's outset, you should embody calmness, serenity, and connection. Your eyes should sparkle with curiosity towards the group, which you regulate with your nervous system and allow yourself to be regulated by in turn, fostering reciprocal attunement. You should motivate and engage participants, illustrating the extraordinary journey of discovery that awaits them and describing its final destination: the reappropriation of their bodies. This is where the autonomic nervous system's activation can best be felt. As an instructor, you must instill confidence in the possibility of change. The body can transform from merely the target of limiting physical symptoms and unpleasant states of activation or shut down into the driving force behind a newfound well-being.

Learning Goals

- Understanding the origins and general principles of Polyvagal Theory.
- Learning about the organization and functioning of the nervous system.
- Exploring the connection between the nervous system's responses to certain stimuli and the relationships experienced with attachment figures during childhood.

Session Framework

1 Welcome, rules of conduct, and session opening – 30 minutes
2 Introductions – 40 minutes
3 Polyvagal Module 1 – 60 minutes
4 Setting homework – 10 minutes
5 Closing ritual and farewell – 10 minutes

N.B.: The times indicated – for this session and those that follow – are only intended as a guide. The process should be adapted to the group's needs, which we encourage you to prioritize as part of your roadmap.

DOI: 10.4324/9781003560968-6

1.1   Welcome, Rules of Conduct, and Session Opening

The instructor begins by introducing themself and welcoming the group. Once the ice has been broken and a warm atmosphere established, lay down some general rules of behavior, being sure to cover:

- The importance of arriving on time.
- The need to provide prior notice for any inability to attend.
- The necessity of ensuring privacy and confidentiality, emphasizing that any information shared during the sessions must not be disclosed outside the group.
- The expectation that homework will be completed and the relevant worksheets submitted on time (within four days of the session) via e-mail or a dedicated messaging group.
- The understanding that homework will be shared with the group. If a participant has an issue with this, they should be invited to discuss it privately with the instructor. Remember that confidentiality is not only a legal requirement, but also a cornerstone of building trust.

Take a moment also to discuss how you want participants to communicate with each other, opening up to mutual polyvagal attunement. Encourage them to share their experiences without interrupting others, giving suggestions, expressing criticism, or offering reassurance. Invite them to listen to one another with genuine, focused attention and an open heart. This way, all experiences will serve as a source of inspiration and growth for everyone in the group.

Remind participants that some activities may be emotionally challenging, and encourage the group to prioritize self-care. If an exercise triggers overwhelming discomfort, they should take time out. In cases like this, stopping to make herbal tea or splash water on one's face is advisable. Such moments are excellent opportunities to practice breathing as a regulating tool, inhaling deeply and exhaling slowly. Ensure participants know to come to you if they cannot manage their feelings or responses independently. If the program is conducted online, make clear they can use the private messaging function for this type of communication.

Here is an example script for your opening speech. Feel free to modify it to suit your own style:

> Good morning everyone. My name is (*your name*), I am pleased to welcome you to the departure station of this extraordinary journey that we are about to embark upon together. Our itinerary includes a series of stops, each linked to the next, leading us to our final destination: awareness of our autonomic nervous system, understanding its profound wisdom, and acquiring tools to begin interacting with it. We will reclaim our bodies. They will no longer be adversaries, but rather the temple of our well-being.

> It is possible that some of you are feeling emotional right now, perhaps slightly anxious or even completely detached. All of this is perfectly normal. Since we don't know each other yet, your nervous system is attempting to determine whether you feel safe here, among these people.
>
> We will now take a few minutes to establish some ground rules of conduct to safeguard ourselves and our learning environment. These guidelines serve as a protective fence around our space, helping to foster a calm and respectful atmosphere where everyone can feel at ease.

Continue by outlining the rules of conduct.

1.2   Introductions

At this point, participants should be invited to briefly introduce themselves, share what they wish to disclose, explain their reasons for joining the program, and articulate what they hope to gain from it. How long each individual's contribution should take will depend on the group size. As the instructor, monitor the time carefully to ensure not to exceed 40 minutes overall.

1.3   Polyvagal Module 1

As explained in Chapter 3, the theoretical concepts in each Module should be presented in a captivating and engaging manner, with ample use of visual aids.

In this first session, the instructor introduces the origins of Polyvagal Theory, explains the vagus nerve, and identifies its path within the body. Following this is an overview of the nervous system's general structure. To this end, you can use the diagrams and images available for download in color from the online resources accompanying this book.

Here is a sample script showing how this information may be presented:

> As I mentioned, our polyvagal journey unfolds in a series of stages. The first stage involves understanding how our extraordinary nervous system is organized. Knowing our biological structure will help illuminate the reasons behind some of our bodily responses – responses that can determine how we feel and even how we think.
>
> Our biology underpins our well-being and discomfort. By understanding how it operates, you will begin to orient yourself within the physiological processes that shape your experience moment by moment.

As previously explained, Polyvagal Theory has revolutionized the classical binary model of the autonomic nervous system, which typically divides it into sympathetic and parasympathetic (Figure 1.1). After presenting this concept, the instructor will

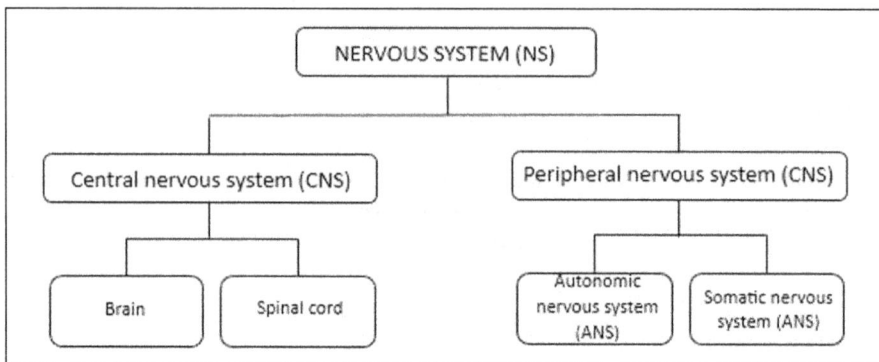

Figure 1.1 The Central and Peripheral Nervous Systems.

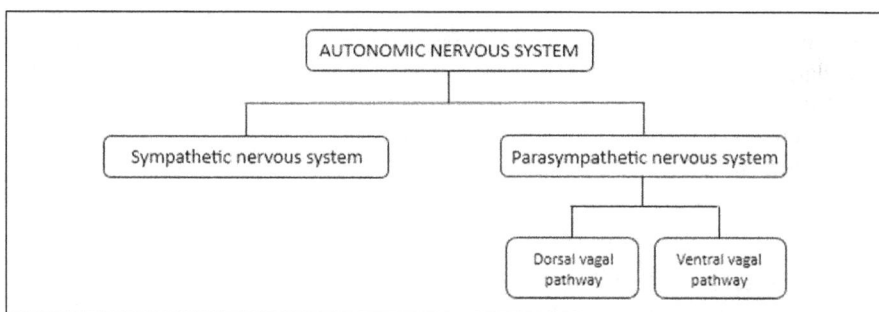

Figure 1.2 The Autonomic Nervous System.

elaborate on how Porges redefined the architecture of this system into three components (Figure 1.2):

- Ventral vagal.
- Sympathetic.
- Dorsal vagal.

This new map of the nervous system, with its specific functional characteristics, can be introduced using the image of the Polyvagal House (Figure 1.3). Let us see how:

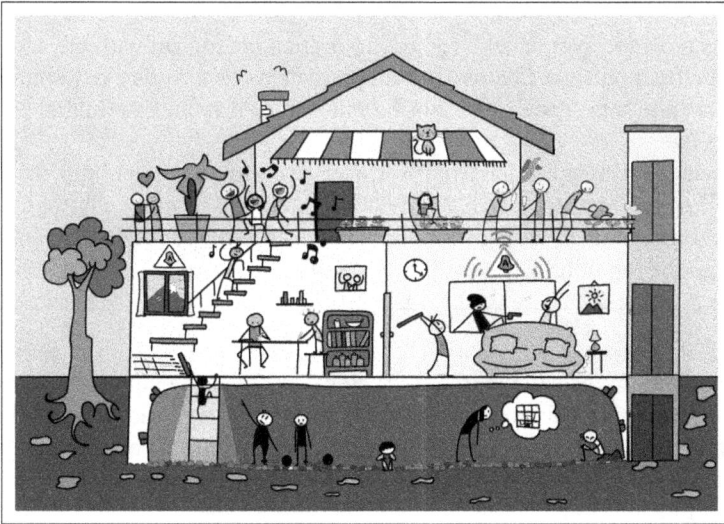

Figure 1.3 The Polyvagal House: A Visual Representation of the Autonomic Nervous System.

Picture your autonomic nervous system (ANS) as a house with three stories: a basement, a first floor with two rooms, and an upper floor.

Look at the first floor. The room on the left represents our ANS in balance. In this room, we feel serene. We can work and carry out everyday tasks with ease. In contrast, the room on the right symbolizes our sympathetic nervous system. We retreat to this room when the alarm has sounded and we sense danger, prompting us to fight or flee (mobilization).

Here, we experience anxiety, fear, sweating, a racing heart, and tense muscles. Although these emotions and physical sensations can be uncomfortable, they are natural responses to perceived threats. They tell us that our nervous system is functioning as it should.

Now, look at the basement. This exemplifies our dorsal vagal system. When we are down there, we don't seem to have a way out. We feel trapped and hopeless, and what is happening to us is so overwhelming that we shut down – essentially, we are playing possum. Our minds go blank, and we are lost for words. Our only option is to freeze (immobilization).

Now to the top floor. This symbolizes our ventral vagal system. When we are up there, we feel safe, calm, and at peace, allowing us to connect with ourselves, others, and our surroundings. We can enjoy the beauty of life – friends, music, plants, kittens, love – anything that brings us joy. Wouldn't it be wonderful to remain here all the time?

However, in response to the signals of safety or danger that we perceive in our surroundings, in the people around us, and within ourselves, we move from one part of the house to the others. Where we go is dictated by our nervous system. If a threat is detected and our ANS judges that we can cope, it directs us to the sympathetic room. If our attempts to deal with the situation through fight or flight fail, our system protects us by ushering us to the basement. While this space might not be much fun, it requires minimal energy to survive.

Once the danger has passed, if we want to return to the top floor, we must ascend to the first floor and spend some time there to gradually regain our equilibrium. Only by doing so will we gather the energy needed to climb the stairs to the top floor, where serenity and openness await.

At this point in the session, the instructor introduces the concept that our autonomic responses are habitual and forged during our early years. You will explain why some individuals predominantly experience a state of alarm or shutdown, even in the absence of objective threats to their safety. Below is an example of how to present this idea to the group.

It should now be clear that our feelings, bodily reactions, emotions, and thoughts in certain situations depend on how our nervous system responds to specific stimuli. You should also understand that our autonomic nervous system acts to protect us.

So, why do some of us spend most of our time in a constant state of alarm, struggling to stay calm? Why do others feel mostly disconnected, detached, and excluded from life, which they see flowing past them as if under glass?

Well, each of us is born with an incredibly plastic nervous system: our ANS can be molded by our experiences. Right from the womb, what happens to us – the atmosphere in our home and the way our caregivers interact with, talk to, and reassure us – shapes how we respond to adversity (Figure 1.4).

Our early experiences sculpt us, much like the potter's hands fashion clay. The way we tend to respond to the many stimuli we come into contact with every day depends heavily on our early interactions. Our history influences the "instruction manual" that our nervous system uses to determine how and when to activate. If we grow up in a strict, threatening, violent, insecure, neglectful, or unpredictable environment, we may feel under constant threat, even when we should feel safe. Consequently, we may find ourselves endlessly mobilized for fight or flight or, conversely, unable to mobilize the energy to defend ourselves, even when it would be appropriate or necessary.

This program is designed to help you understand why your nervous system responds as it does to certain stimuli. Step by step, we will work together to construct a new biological platform – a new instruction manual for your ANS – that will empower you to lead a healthier, happier life.

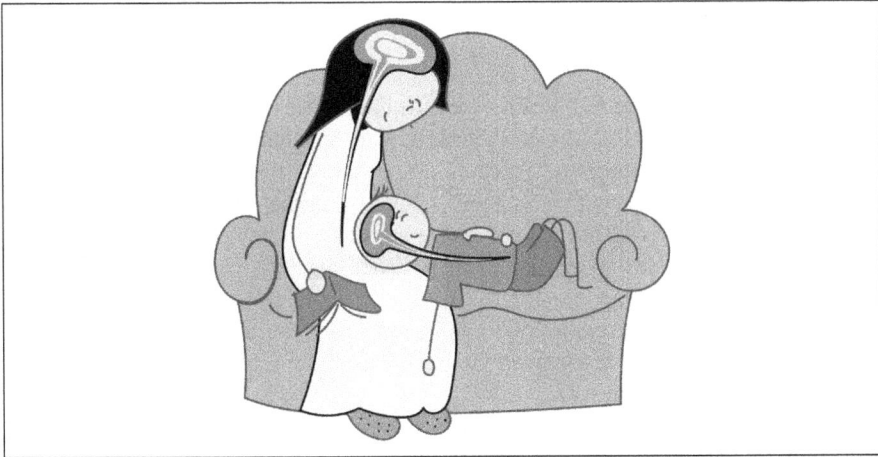

Figure 1.4 Our Early Experiences of Relationships Shape the Responses of Our Autonomic Nervous System.

1.4 Setting Homework

Cultivate Awareness: Your Early Relationship Experiences

In this part of the session, the instructor introduces the homework for the week. This is an excellent opportunity to emphasize the importance of homework as an essential aspect of the learning process. Confirm that all participants understand the theoretical concepts presented, and address any questions or uncertainties they may have. Since the homework is closely related to the module content, reiterating key points will help ensure the material has been grasped. Introduce the homework assignment as follows:

How our autonomic nervous system responds to certain stimuli reflects our relationship experiences during our early years. Take some time to reflect on your childhood, and your relationships with your primary caregivers (mother, father, etc.). Write down your answers to the following questions:

- Did you grow up with reassuring, calm, emotionally available caregivers? Or were they anxious, cold, angry, distant, or unpredictable?
- How would you characterize your overall experience?
- Which of your caregivers do you believe has had the greatest impact on you?
- How do you think these experiences have affected your nervous system?

1.5   Closing Ritual and Farewell

The Power of Breath: Breathing Out

The instructor concludes the session by introducing the first experiential exercise of the course. The goal is to allow the group to familiarize themselves with the learning model of the program, which combines theory with practice. This activity is designed to guide the participants into a state of regulation, so they can begin to experience the beneficial impact of simple actions on their own nervous system. Lead them through it using the following instructions:

- Sit in a comfortable position, feet planted firmly on the floor and your back straight but relaxed, away from the backrest of your chair.
- Turn your attention inward.
- Take five short, light breaths in, each followed by a long breath out.
- Keep your abdomen relaxed, especially as you exhale.

At the end of five breathing cycles, ask participants to notice the effect of the exercise on their body. How do they feel now?

Conclude the session by expressing gratitude for the nervous systems of all participants and extend a collective farewell. Encourage them to pay attention to their autonomic responses as often as possible until the next session.

Session 2

The Key Principles of Polyvagal Theory

In this meeting, the instructor should continue to foster a sense of safety and connection within the group. Be attentive, curious, warm, and welcoming, and make a determined and consistent effort to create a polyvagal atmosphere in the classroom. This session marks the first occasion for participants to share their homework in front of others – a crucial moment in which individuals begin to open up, share personal stories, and reveal their inner world. From this reciprocal disclosure, the seeds of positive relationships start taking root.

This session also introduces the first cardinal principles of Polyvagal Theory. The concepts presented are foundational and will serve as a reference framework throughout the entire journey. Consequently, the content will be dense, making this meeting the most intellectually demanding of the entire program. While these principles will be revisited and consolidated in future classes, it is in this session that the basic building blocks of the Polyvagal House will be assembled. The theory discussed in this module is complemented by a guided imagery activity, allowing the group to develop a visceral understanding of their autonomic states. Participants are preparing to become experts in their nervous systems on both cognitive and embodied levels.

Learning Goals

- Gaining a deeper understanding of the connection between habitual nervous system responses and early life experiences through group sharing of homework.
- Understanding the three key principles of Polyvagal Theory: autonomic hierarchy, neuroception, and co-regulation.
- Developing awareness of one's autonomic landscape and its three sections: ventral vagal, sympathetic, and dorsal vagal.

Session Framework

1 Session opening and homework review – 60 minutes
2 Polyvagal Module 2 – 60 minutes

DOI: 10.4324/9781003560968-7

3   Experiential learning: guided imagery – 30 minutes
4   Setting homework – 10 minutes
5   Closing ritual and farewell – 5 minutes

N.B.: The times indicated are only intended as a guide. The process should be adapted to the group's needs, which we encourage you to prioritize as part of your roadmap.

2.1   Session Opening and Homework Review

After welcoming everyone to the group, the instructor leads the sharing of the previous session's homework. Ensure you read all participants' contributions beforehand to facilitate a smooth exchange. Invite each person to present their work, one by one. If necessary, follow up with a moment of deeper exploration with each individual and continue the practice in future meetings. It is important to note that this open discussion of homework can leave people feeling exposed and vulnerable. Communicating with the group in a compassionate, kind, and respectful manner – as outlined in Chapter 2 – is crucial to creating a warm, safe, and welcoming environment. Approach the experiences reported with curiosity and avoid any form of judgment. This way, you will transform the homework review into a springboard for further discussion of concepts and an opportunity to cultivate meaningful connections among you and the individuals in the group. Remind them to listen actively without commenting. Encourage them to open up their autonomic nervous systems to the experiences of others and to view these with sensitivity and an open mind. As always, group sharing is an opportunity for everyone to learn from each other's insights.

2.2   Polyvagal Module 2

In this second meeting, the instructor presents the three cardinal principles of Polyvagal Theory: autonomic hierarchy, neuroception, and co-regulation. In the previous session, we outlined the structure and function of the autonomic nervous system using the Polyvagal House. Today, we will explore another metaphor borrowed from Dana (2018, p. 10): the Autonomic Ladder (Figure 2.1).

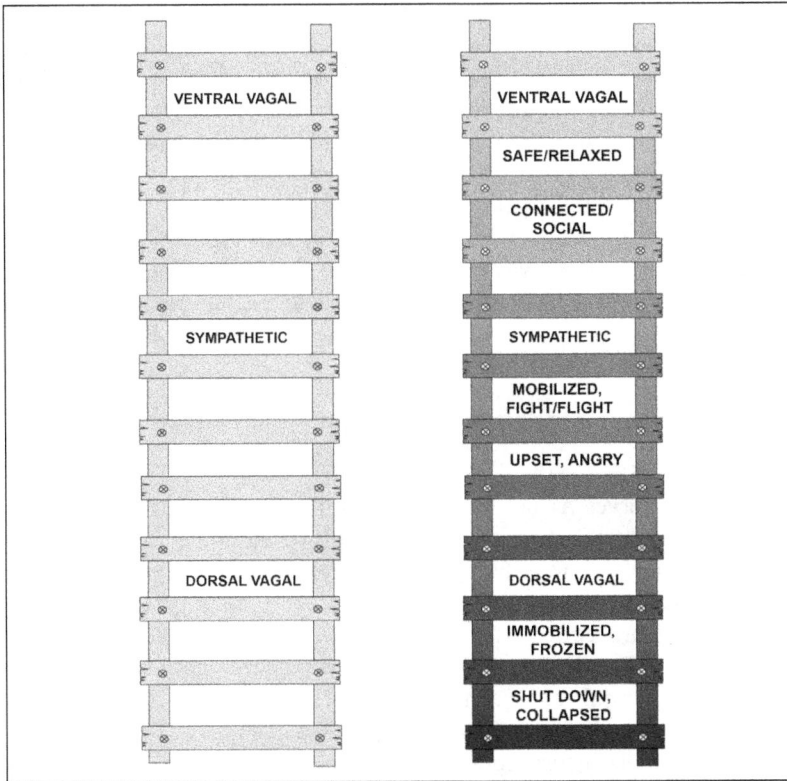

Figure 2.1 The Autonomic Ladder according to Deb Dana.

From *The Polyvagal Theory in Therapy: Engaging the Rhythm of Regulation* by Deb Dana. Copyright © 2018 by Deb Dana. Used by permission of W. W. Norton & Company, Inc.

In our first meeting, we began familiarizing ourselves with the autonomic nervous system through the image of the Polyvagal House. Do you remember its floors and rooms? Can you recall how we feel in each space and why we move from one environment to another?

Today, we will use the ladder metaphor to illustrate one of the key elements of Polyvagal Theory: the autonomic hierarchy, and how the various sections of the nervous system interconnect. As you can see, the ladder's lower rungs represent the dorsal vagal state, the middle section indicates the sympathetic, and the upper part reflects the ventral vagal.

Throughout our day, our autonomic nervous system guides us up and down this ladder, transitioning between states, through various nuances.

When we feel calm and safe, we dwell in a state of balance. The upper rungs of the ladder represent multiple levels at which we can experience harmony and connection with ourselves and the world, culminating in a profound sense of happiness, being blessed.

However, when faced with a problem, an obstacle, or a triggering thought that sets off our internal alarms, we start slipping down the ladder. We find ourselves on the sympathetic rungs and may plunge even lower, into the dorsal vagal state, if we feel that the issue is too much to cope with. We must learn to recognize where we are on the ladder at any given moment. Only by doing so can we modulate our emotional state and achieve a sense of safety and connection.

Next, go on to illustrate the principle of neuroception using the metaphor of antennas.

Neuroception serves as our personal surveillance system. It continuously monitors our internal states, the surrounding environment, and the people around us, often without us being aware. When a potential threat is detected, the alarm sounds, triggering our bodies to prepare for action or shut down completely. Neuroception's primary question is: "Am I safe here?" If the answer is yes, we can remain at the top of the ladder – or on the top floor of the house – in ventral vagal safety. If the answer is no, we go down to a lower rung where we can better defend or protect ourselves.

We can visualize neuroception as a set of exceptionally sensitive antennas that we all possess. These antennas continuously track a multitude of signals that reach us during the day. Although the illustrations in this book only show antennas on the head, it's important to remember that our entire bodies, and all of our senses, are standing watch. In the previous meeting, we explored how early experiences shape our autonomic nervous system's responses. In doing so, these experiences actually construct our neuroception, they build our antennas. This explains why our neuroception may not always provide accurate information. Sometimes, the alarm is triggered by objectively threatening events – a fire or a robbery – while other times we respond to our internal perception of reality, for example, when we feel uncomfortable in our bodies or experience crushing insecurity at a party full of people we don't know (Figure 2.2).

The final part of the module addresses co-regulation. Explain its biological foundation as follows:

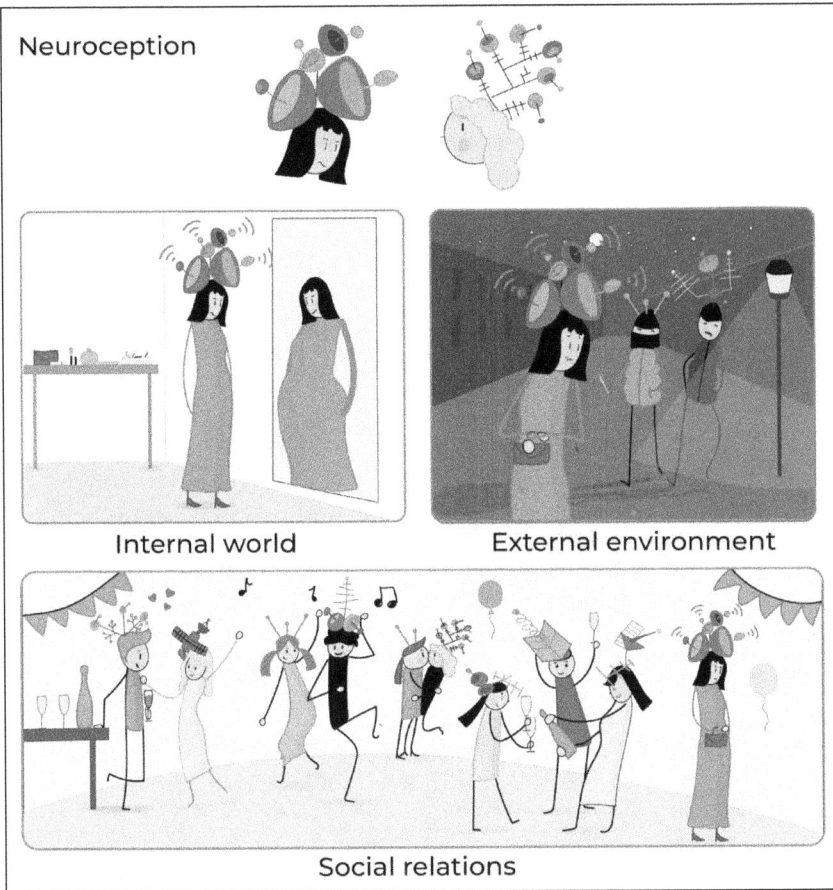

Figure 2.2 Neuroception Acts without Our Conscious Control. Our nervous system is constantly scanning our body and internal world, our external environment, and the people around us for signals of safety or danger.

We enter the world as amazing but weak and vulnerable beings, reliant on adults to nurture us to reach our inherent potential. This need for calm, relaxation, and regulation through others accompanies us from the day we are born and remains an integral part of us throughout the course of our life. Our nervous systems connect and synchronize through an intricate dance involving eye contact, the voice, heart rate, and breathing. Think of locking eyes with a close friend, or even a new acquaintance, at a dinner table while they are telling a captivating story; chances are, you are experiencing an unspoken understanding of each other's thoughts and feelings, resulting in a shared smile that uplifts you both.

This process, in which bodies, minds, and hearts unite, is called co-regulation. We need others. We need positive and long-lasting relationships.

Connection safeguards our health and promotes our well-being. Our bonds of love are essential not only during childhood but also for our psychological and physical equilibrium as adults. In some way, the need for co-regulation makes us all alike and dependent on each other: each of us offers co-regulation and receives co-regulation in return (Figure 2.3).

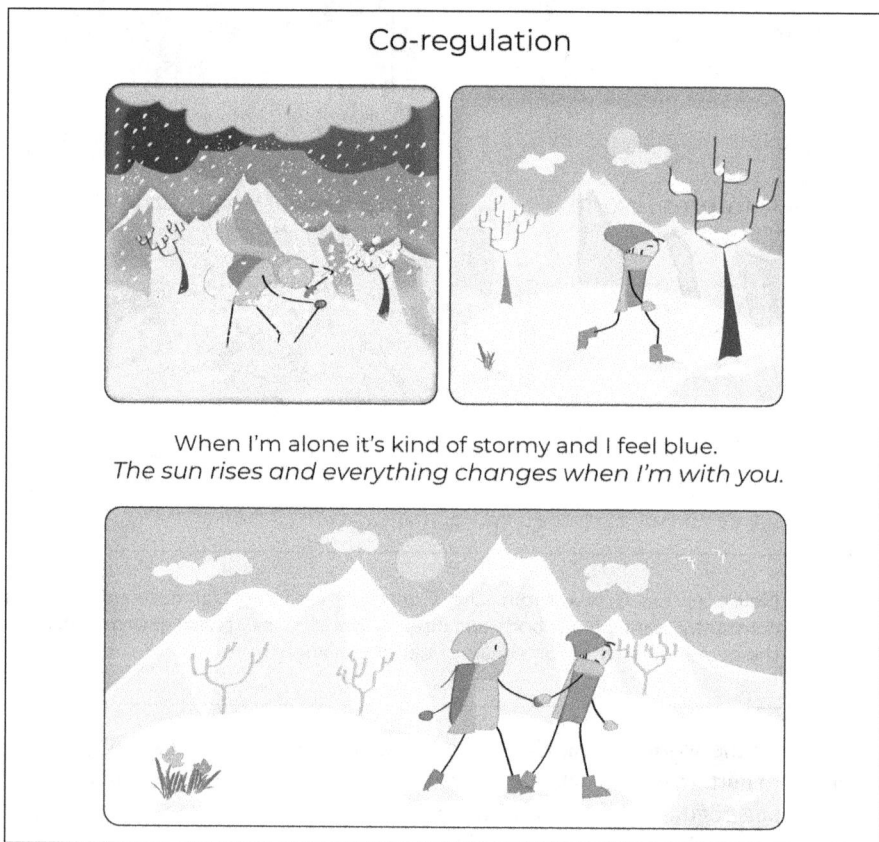

Co-regulation

When I'm alone it's kind of stormy and I feel blue.
The sun rises and everything changes when I'm with you.

Figure 2.3 Co-regulation: A Biological Imperative.

2.3   Experiential Learning: Guided Imagery

Befriending Your Autonomic Nervous System

This exercise marks the first time participants will engage in guided imagery. Therefore, it's essential to provide preliminary instructions to help everyone immerse themselves and derive meaning from the activity. Begin by briefly explaining that, during guided imagery, we should direct our attention inward, observing our experiences as they unfold, embracing them without judgment. This practice will allow us to understand our autonomic landscape, how our bodies react, what emotions we feel, and how we think in different states of activation.

Posture is important. Participants should be comfortable and relaxed, yet attentive. Encourage them to:

- Sit on the front of their chair seat.
- Plant their feet firmly on the ground.
- Place their hands, relaxed, on their thighs.
- Maintain an upright posture with their neck straight and shoulders gently opened, aligning them, as well as possible, with their pelvis.

If any participant struggles with this position, encourage them to adjust it for comfort, using cushions or rolled towels as needed. The goal is to be free of any tension or pain that could get in the way of their experience. Emphasize the importance of knowing their limits and practicing self-care.

Once you have ensured everyone is ready and in the correct position, you can begin leading the guided imagery activity using the script below. You do not need to read it word for word or learn it by heart. Think of it merely as a guide you can adapt to the group's needs as you become more confident. Provide participants with a pre-recorded audio file to practice this exercise at home, allowing them to absorb the insights fully.

Imagine a lighthouse. Turn that light of awareness upon yourself. Let your attention rest on your breathing for a while. Breathe in and out consciously, focusing on the sensations evoked as you do so.

(Pause for a few seconds)

Imagine now that you are near the top of your ladder, in the ventral vagal state. You feel safe and relaxed and are enjoying the view. Bask in this calming energy for a few seconds by thinking about the last time you felt truly good, safe, peaceful, and serene. In your mind's eye, try to relive that experience fully. Notice the details: Where are you? What are you doing? Who are you with?

(Pause for a few seconds)

Stay there for a while. How do you feel? How do your muscles respond? What is happening to your breathing? And your heart rate? What kind of emotions arise? What kind of thoughts come to mind? Spend some time studying yourself, gathering information about your ventral vagal state.

(Pause for a few seconds)

Allow that image to fade and return to the here and now, focusing on your breath for a moment.

Now, go down a step, into the activation and mobilization energy of your sympathetic nervous system. Think of a situation that triggers some anxiety but is manageable, such as a pot boiling over or the worry of potentially missing a bus. Your goal is to observe your reactions in such situations.

(Pause for a few seconds)

Immerse yourself in the sympathetic state for a while… What is happening in your body? What sensations do you feel? How are your breath and heart responding? Does your overall energy change? If so, how? Perhaps you feel an urge to move or take action… What is that impulse? What emotions arise? What thoughts emerge? Take some time to gather information.

(Pause for a few seconds)

Now, transition away from your sympathetic state using your breathing to return to ventral vagal regulation… If you wish, you can try to exhale for longer than you inhale. Keep your belly soft as you breathe in, then breathe out slowly. Breathing this way is your ticket back home, your route back to the warmth and safety of ventral vagal regulation.

(Pause for a few seconds)

Finally, imagine going further down the ladder into your dorsal vagal state. Remember that there is no need to be alarmed: this is merely a fact-finding mission. You are intentionally venturing into the deeper parts of your autonomic nervous system, but you can stop at any point on the ladder. Think of a circumstance where you felt a little upset, closed off, or withdrawn from everyone and everything. Perhaps a friend didn't call when they said they would, or you made a mistake at work. Immerse yourself in that situation. Stay there for a while. Now, notice what happens to your body…

(Pause for a few seconds)

How is your breathing? How does your heart react? Study your overall energy. Does it change? What emotions do you feel? What kind of thoughts arise? Gather insights about your dorsal vagal state.

(Pause for a few seconds)

Now, consciously climb up the ladder. Take time to remind yourself no threat or danger is happening now. If you need to ground yourself, press your feet to the floor or push your hands against each other for a few moments. Use your breath to gradually climb the rungs back to the top. Keep your belly soft, inhaling and exhaling slowly. This way of breathing is your anchor; it acts as a lifeline, allowing you to return to the calm sea of ventral vagal regulation.

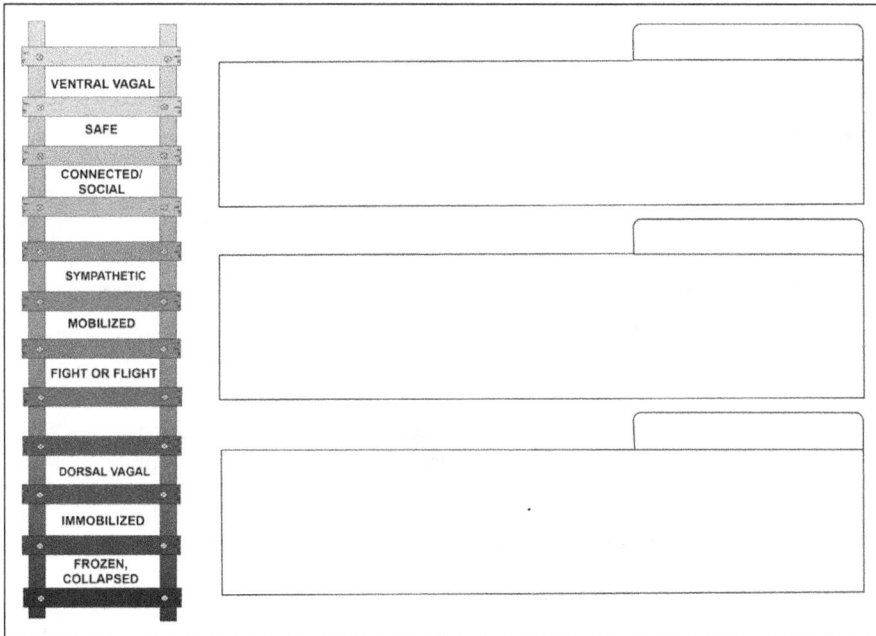

Figure 2.4 Personal Profile Map.

From *The Polyvagal Theory in Therapy: Engaging the Rhythm of Regulation* by Deb Dana. Copyright © 2018 by Deb Dana. Used by permission of W. W. Norton & Company, Inc.

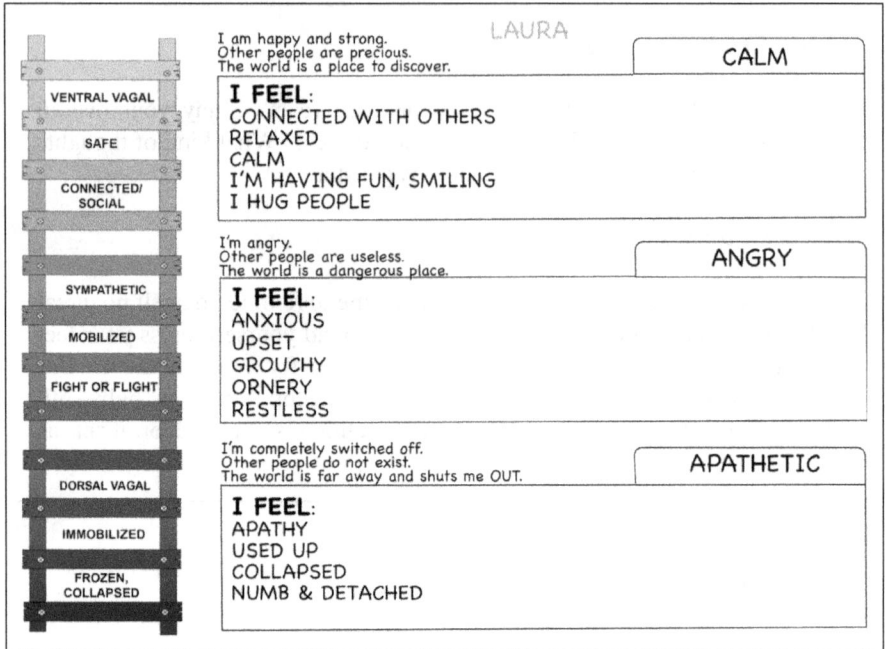

Figure 2.5 An Example Personal Profile Map Filled Out for Homework.

2.4   Setting Homework

Personal Profile Map

In this phase, the instructor introduces assignments for the upcoming week, following the guidelines previously provided. The group will complete the Personal Profile Map (Dana 2018, p. 59), an example of which, filled out by a course participant, is provided above (Figure 2.5).

During the guided imagery exercise, you gained a clearer understanding of your autonomic states. Returning to that experience, fill out your Personal Profile Map as follows:

- Choose a color for each state – ventral vagal, sympathetic, and dorsal vagal.
- Describe how you feel in each state. Happy? Sad? Joyful? Afraid? Describe your body sensations, emotions, thoughts, and actions in each state.
- Choose a keyword that sums up the essence of each state.

- Complete the following sentences for each state, beginning with dorsal vagal, then sympathetic, and finally ventral vagal:
  - I am…
  - Others are…
  - The world is…

If you like, decorate the boxes with the colors you have chosen. Feel free to draw pictures or use emojis that represent how you feel.

2.5   Closing Ritual and Farewell

The group has just concluded their first exploration of guided imagery after a content-rich session; for this reason, the closing ritual simply consists of three calming breaths in and out (see the instructions in Session 1).

End the meeting by expressing gratitude to the nervous systems of all participants, encouraging them to remain attuned to their autonomic responses as often as possible, and a collective farewell.

Session 3

Lights, Shadows, and Bridges

The group is beginning to coalesce. Participants are mastering polyvagal terminology. At this point, they will have embraced the concept of *autonomic activation*. They now understand how this phenomenon affects their physiology and, consequently, their emotional experiences, governing their impulses to act and the thoughts they tend to produce when in a certain state. The focus of this session is to help them familiarize themselves with their own triggers and discover what their neuroception interprets as danger or safety signals.

Learning Goals

- Gaining more insight into the three branches of the autonomic nervous system through group sharing of homework.
- Beginning to recognize situations that elicit specific reactions and consciously utilize this knowledge.
- Understanding the connection between personal triggers and autonomic responses.

Session Framework

1. Session opening and homework review – 60 minutes
2. Polyvagal Module 3 – 30 minutes
3. Experiential learning: mapping Lights and Shadows – 50 minutes
4. Setting homework: Bridges – 15 minutes
5. Closing ritual and farewell – 10 minutes

N.B.: The times indicated are only intended as a guide. The process should be adapted to the group's needs, which we encourage you to prioritize as part of your roadmap.

3.1 Session Opening and Homework Review

After warmly welcoming the participants, the instructor briefly summarizes the previous session and conducts the homework review, following the guidelines previously provided.

DOI: 10.4324/9781003560968-8

3.2 Polyvagal Module 3

Today's session introduces the powerful concept of *Lights* and *Shadows*. *Lights* represent all those events that illuminate our lives, infused with the bright energy of the ventral vagal state – think of a playful puppy, a heartfelt hug, or a friendly wave. In contrast, *Shadows* are those experiences that, like dark clouds, cast a pall over our day – an overdue bill, a flat tire, or a rude cashier. Both Lights and Shadows evoke neuroceptive alerts within us. Lights signal safety, while Shadows convey danger. These triggers guide us up and down the Autonomic Ladder, or from one floor of the Polyvagal House to another.

The next exercise will involve participants mapping their Lights and Shadows. Take time to reiterate that charting the functioning of our autonomic nervous system is a valuable tool for self-awareness. By recognizing their Lights and Shadows, participants can gain insight into their individual reactions. This realization is the first and most crucial step in learning how to move from one state to another.

Imagine you are about to explore a new city. Wouldn't it be wise to have a guide, or at least a map, so you can get around without losing your way?

As we have already said, we too are on a journey. Our destination is getting our autonomic nervous system to work for us rather than against us. We have already completed the initial stages of this exciting itinerary together. The homework we discussed earlier laid the groundwork – the first map of our autonomic landscape allows us to pinpoint where we are on the ladder.

Today, we will introduce another mapping system that will help us decode the language of neuroception and start modifying its basic grammar. We call it the Map of Lights and Shadows (adapted from Dana, 2018, p. 68–69).

But what exactly do we mean by Shadows?

They are the triggers that our nervous system perceives as danger signals, activating our sympathetic or dorsal vagal defense responses.

And what about Lights?

These events are perceived as safety signals. They can lead us up to the warm and quiet energy of the ventral vagal state. Lights help us feel good, they are a balm for our body and soul.

When Lights manifest as small, fleeting moments of well-being scattered throughout the day – sparks of happiness here and there – we refer to them as "glimmers" (Dana, 2020, p. 108). Why do glimmers matter? The experience of positive emotion, even when it lasts for an eyeblink, is still a valuable resource. By learning to focus on these joyful moments, and training ourselves to savor them, they can become significant enough to take us up our Autonomic Ladder. A collection of glimmers can transform into a "glow", a radiant light that brightens our day and alters its hue (Figure 3.1).

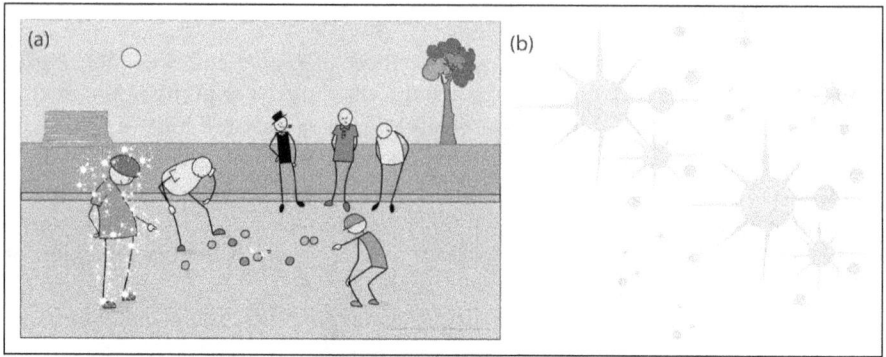

Figure 3.1 A and B Glimmers: Micro-Moments of Well-Being Sprinkled through the Day.

3.3   Experiential Learning

The Map of Lights and Shadows

At this point, guide participants in creating their own Maps of Lights and Shadows (Dana, 2018, p. 69) (Figure 3.2). Provide the following instructions:

- Begin by filling in the various sections, identifying the events or triggers that can plunge you into each autonomic state. Be thorough and take time to reflect

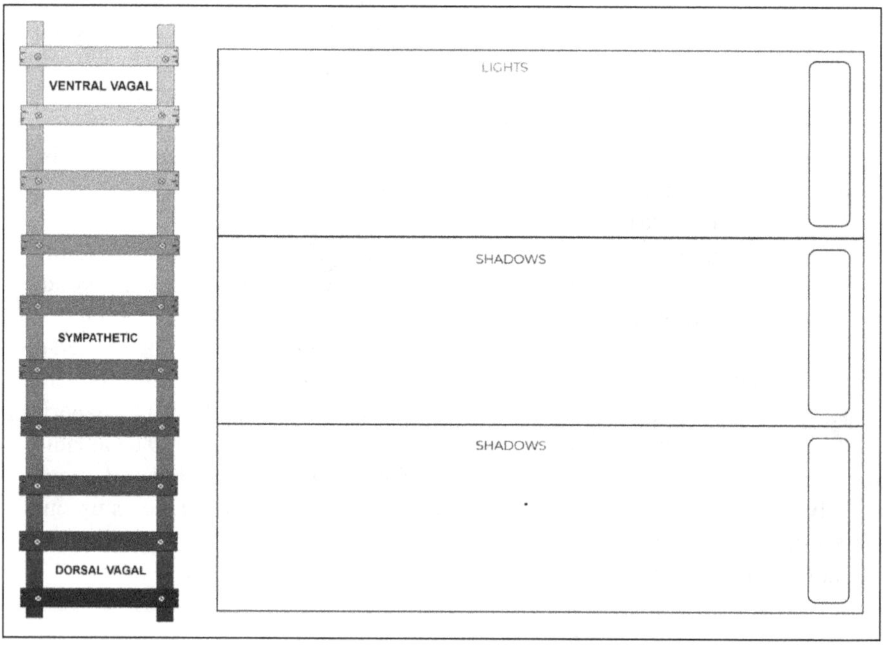

Figure 3.2 Map of Lights and Shadows.

From *The Polyvagal Theory in Therapy: Engaging the Rhythm of Regulation* by Deb Dana. Copyright © 2018 by Deb Dana. Used by permission of W. W. Norton & Company, Inc.

deeply. Inhabit the state you are focusing on. Try to list as many ideas as possible. Ask yourself: When I end up in this state, what brought me here? How did I get to this place?

• Start with the survival response that feels most familiar to you (whether sympathetic or dorsal vagal), then move on to the next. End with the ventral vagal state. If you wish, choose a different color for each state, one which resonates with its essence.

Before they start, divide the participants into small groups of three or four. If teaching online, this is the perfect time to use "breakout rooms" for focused discussion. We recommend that you allocate 20 minutes for individual mapping and 30 minutes for participants to share their map with the group. Remind everyone to listen with openness and empathy, refraining from commenting on others' experiences. It is, however, valuable for participants to express how someone's sharing resonated with them, such as, "Your Light inspires me because…" or "Hearing you talk about that Shadow touched me deeply and reminded me of when I…".

The activity should last a total of 50 minutes and culminate with the whole class coming together to share insights. As an example, see Figure 3.3, which shows a map completed by one of our participants.

PAULA

VENTRAL VAGAL

LIGHTS

WHEN I FEEL LOVED, HUG MY DAUGHTER, PLAY THE PIANO & COMPOSE
MUSIC, SWIMMING IN THE SEA, LOOKING AFTER MY PLANTS,
MY HUSBAND'S ARM AROUND ME WHILE WATCHING A FILM,
EATING A NICE MEAL OUT,
A FOOT MASSAGE,
A HOT SHOWER

GOOD

SYMPATHETIC

SHADOWS

ARGUING WITH SOMEONE WHO SHOUTS,
AGGRESSIVENESS WHEN SOMEONE IS DISRESPECTFUL,
BEING LATE,
HAVING TOO MUCH TO DO,
WHEN MY DAUGHTER DOESN'T WANT TO GO TO SCHOOL,
TRAFFIC JAMS,
DRIVING IN THE CITY,
OTHER PEOPLE BEING RUDE,
NOT BEING ABLE TO DO SOMETHING

UPSET

DORSAL VAGAL

SHADOWS

ILLNESS AND PHYSICAL PAIN,
WHEN I'M AVOIDANT,
WHEN I FEEL PRETTY WORTHLESS,
IF I GET IGNORED,
LONELINESS,
WALKING
ALONE IN THE DARK,
FEAR OF LOSING SOMEONE I LOVE

GLOOMY

Figure 3.3 An Example Map of Lights and Shadows Filled Out by a Course Participant.

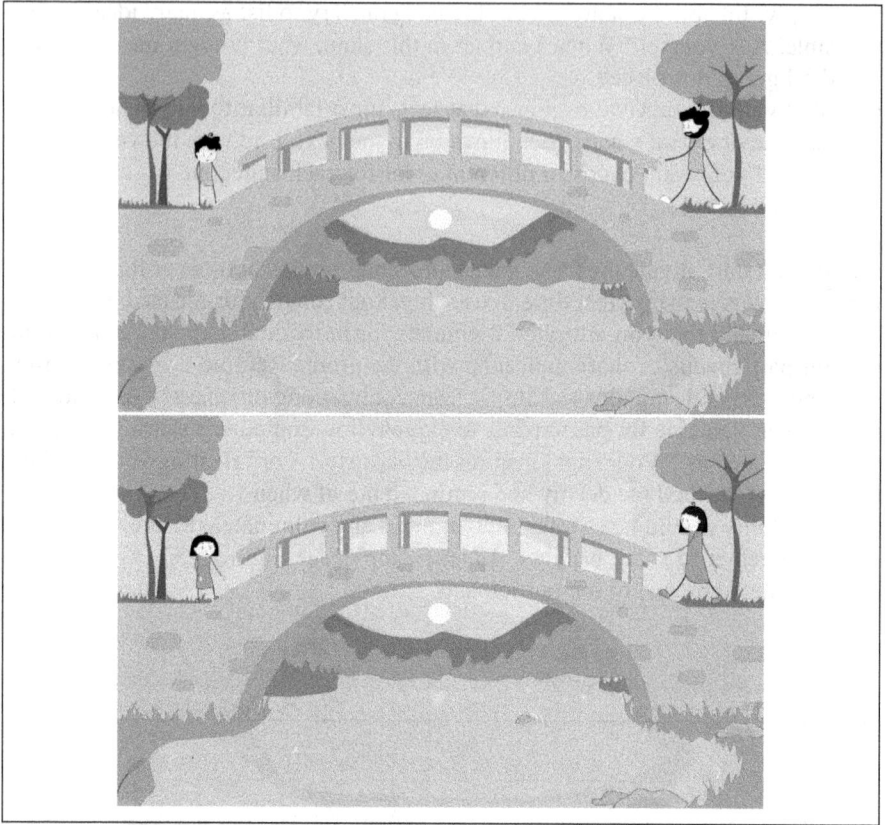

Figure 3.4 There Is Often a Bridge between How Neuroception Responds in the Present and What Happened to Us in the Past.

3.4   Setting Homework

Building a Bridge to the Past

The homework for the week – called "Building a Bridge to the Past" – consists of creating a link between our reactions in the present and the historical circumstances that shaped our autonomic tendencies. You can find examples of this homework filled out by course participants at the end of this section (Figure 3.5 and 3.6). This assignment requires a brief introduction. Here is a script to guide you through the process:

But where do our Shadows come from? Why do some situations or people – a particular tone of voice or a certain gesture – trigger our autonomic nervous system, plunging us into the sympathetic or dorsal vagal state, while others do not?

We passively suffer and endure these states. Our responses to certain triggers seem normal or logical to us. However, as we are beginning to understand, our neuroception is burdened by baggage from the past. Today, we will work on building a bridge to that past, exploring the link between what happened to us *then* and how we react *now*.

THERESA

This has been my reality since I was a child, and it still persists. Around food, the sympathetic (ambivalent) pathway is activated—mainly with anger, because I can't control myself, and anxiety, because I feel like I should be able to control myself. When I fail, I enter the dorsal vagal state. I feel like I am nothing and shut myself off. I can't shake the painful emotional legacy around food that my family gave me.

This internal battle happens almost every day. It's definitely a bridge to the past. Even though I no longer live with my father, I have now been continuing the same cycle for 10 years. When I was little, my father—and then the rest of the family—made me feel bad about myself and my body. He was always saying (even though it wasn't objectively true) that I was "overweight" or that I had acne. These comments, his expressions of contempt, and my compulsive dieting made me feel inadequate, ugly, and angry. I felt angry with myself because I could never be thin and pretty enough. I would put myself through painful scrutiny and end up feeling weak and spineless because I could never stick to a diet—even though I didn't have to.

MARK

I'm at the park with my son; while he is playing, a child bites him on the cheek. My dorsal vagal activates. Bridge: my teacher, in the first grade, slaps my classmate. I feel totally hopeless and freeze.

Figure 3.5 Bridges: Examples of Homework Assignments Completed by Course Participants.

Present the task by providing these instructions:

- Think of a recent event that plunged you into a sympathetic or dorsal vagal state.
- Focus your attention inward and immerse yourself in the bodily sensations, emotions, and thoughts evoked by that situation. If you wish, jot down words that describe your internal world.

- Give yourself time to reflect and try to build a bridge to your past. Does what you feel today remind you of a moment from childhood when you experienced something similar?
- Document your insights as you build your bridge (Figure 3.4). How are your current reactions somehow connected to what happened at that time?

3.5   Closing Ritual and Farewell

Posture and Gaze

The session concludes with an exercise to stimulate the vagus nerve through posture and gaze. Invite participants to follow these instructions (Figure 3.6).

- Cross your hands behind the back of your neck and open your shoulders wide. Remember to be gentle with yourself and respect your limits.
- Keep your head still with your gaze focused forward.
- Look up towards your left eyebrow.
- Hold this position for 10 seconds.
- Slowly rotate your eyes towards the right eyebrow.
- Repeat this sequence three times.

After the exercise, encourage participants to take a moment to reflect on the sensations they feel and the impact of this practice.

Close the meeting by expressing gratitude to the nervous system of all participants. Encourage the group to remain conscious of their autonomic responses throughout their daily lives, and to use breathwork as a regulatory resource whenever possible.

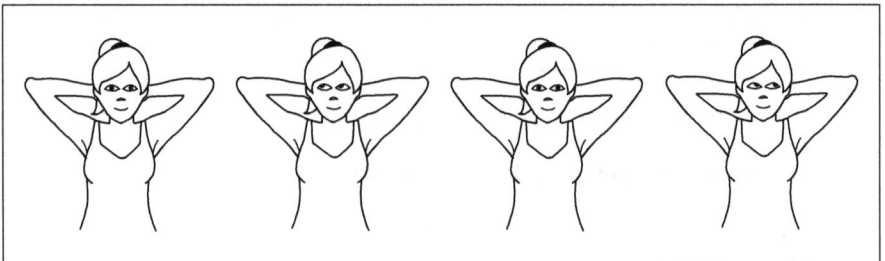

Figure 3.6 The Gaze.

Personal Resources

Participants are beginning to savor a sense of connection within the group. They are becoming more aware of their Lights and Shadows. Their understanding of the events or situations that can catapult them into a certain autonomic state is growing.

In this session, the instructor encourages everyone to take a step further: recognizing the resources they already possess to climb out of sympathetic mobilization and/or dorsal vagal immobilization and return to the soothing embrace of ventral vagal energy. At this stage in their journey, the primary goal of *Wired to Connect* is learning how to interrupt typical autonomic survival responses and to live life from a baseline feeling of safety and regulation.

Learning Goals

- Further understanding the connection between neuroception and personal history through the homework review.
- Recognizing the set of personal resources already present in one's life for shifting out of a certain autonomic state.

Session Framework

1 Session opening and homework review – 50 minutes
2 Polyvagal Module 4 – 30 minutes
3 Experiential learning: guided imagery – 25 minutes
4 Setting homework – 10 minutes
5 Closing ritual and farewell – 10 minutes

N.B.: The times indicated are only intended as a guide. The process should be adapted to the group's needs, which we encourage you to prioritize as part of your roadmap.

DOI: 10.4324/9781003560968-9

4.1   Session Opening and Homework Review

After warmly welcoming the participants, the instructor provides a brief summary of the previous session and proceeds to review the homework. Sharing the "Building a Bridge to the Past" assignment allows the group to cement their understanding that our perception is shaped by our early life experiences, which are beyond our control. This theme is central to the program, and this worksheet is normally a source of deep insight.

It is advisable not to rush this part of the process. However, the time allotted for this learning activity may not be sufficient to listen carefully to everyone. If necessary, consider continuing this homework review in the next class.

This part of the meeting can be closed with a comment as below.

> Building bridges with our past and exploring why and how we shift into a certain autonomic state is crucial. It helps us start a new narrative about ourselves, quieting the jarring sound of that self-critical voice we often hear from within. Instead of asking, "Why do I react like this?" we can begin to ask, "Who am I? What's my story?" It is time for us to stop judging ourselves and instead practice self-acceptance and compassion. We did not create our autonomic responses. They depend on what happened to us long ago, sometimes before we even learned to say our name. Once we can accept what *is*, we open the door to transforming what *will be*.

4.2   Polyvagal Module 4

At this point in the session, the instructor should reiterate the importance of mapping systems and introduce the concept of *individual and interactive resources*. Let us see how.

> We already possess a toolbox of resources for dealing with various situations (Figure 4.1). Often, we use these tools without realizing that they help us regulate our autonomic nervous systems.
>
> Some of these things we do alone. For instance, when feeling anxious or down, some may enjoy a walk in nature, while others might listen to music, engage in sports, or practice yoga or meditation. The list is practically endless and very personal.
>
> Generally, to emerge from a dorsal vagal "freeze", we engage in activities that gradually restore our energy and vitality, such as taking a slow walk that

progressively gets brisker. On the other hand, we might vent excess sympathetic energy through running or working out at the gym (Figure 4.2).

There are also things that we can do with others. Let's not forget that we cannot exist in a vacuum, and we need people around for co-regulation. In a relationship, one body/mind modifies the other. Bonds are to our nervous system what fresh, clean air is to our lungs: oxygen.

However, if we grow up in a dysfunctional environment, our autonomic nervous system tends to overreact, making us prone to avoidance, or defensive behaviors. Hence, the positive relationships we can draw on to regulate ourselves may be few and far between. In such cases, how can we begin reaching out to others, cultivating an autonomic place of serenity and trust?

We can all find that sweet spot from which we can forge relationships and reinforce contact with others without entering self-protection mode. The key is to take small steps towards connection that our nervous system will not perceive as too risky or daring. Start with a wave, a smile, or a kind gesture. This session focuses on increasing awareness of the individual and interactive resources already available to us, enabling us to nurture our nervous system and connect with others.

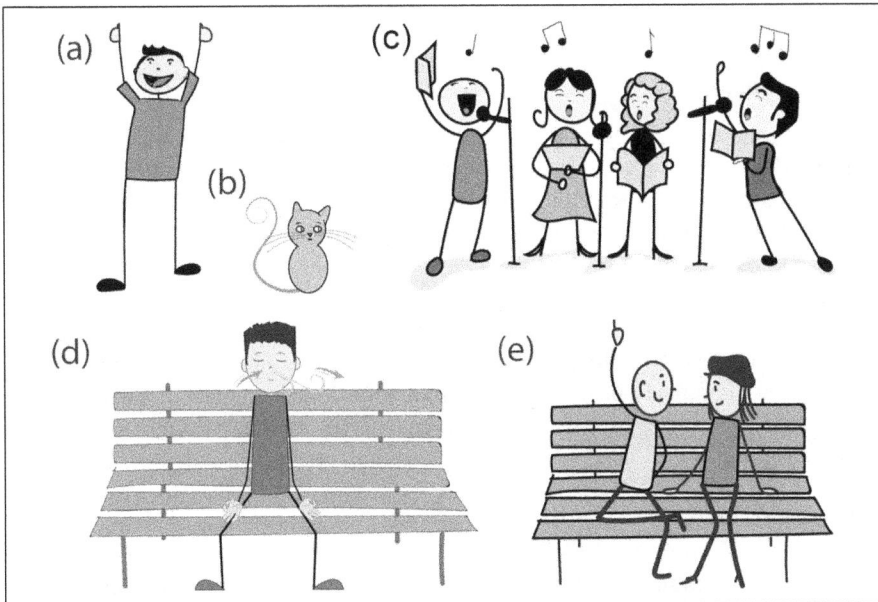

Figure 4.1 (a)–(e) Some Examples of Personal and Interpersonal Resources.

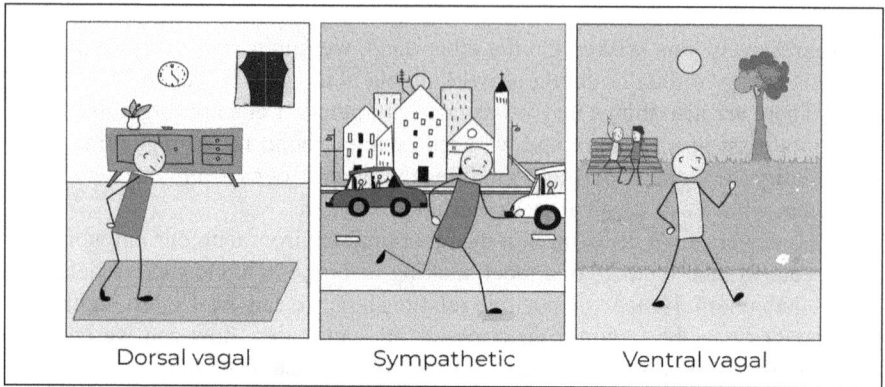

| Dorsal vagal | Sympathetic | Ventral vagal |

Figure 4.2 Modifying Autonomic State by Experimenting with Different Ways of Walking (Slow, Quick, Leisurely).

4.3 Experiential Learning: Guided Imagery

Wired to Connect

As mentioned above, the instructor should create an audio recording of the guided imagery activity before the session. This can be shared with the group for home practice, to enhance their insight. Lead the experience using the same guidelines as in Chapter 2.

Close your eyes gently or keep them slightly open. Alert but relaxed at the same time, observe your experience and embrace it. Enter your inner world by focusing on your breathing for a few cycles. Lengthen each breath. Inhale and exhale slowly while trying to keep your belly relaxed.

(Pause for a few seconds)

When you feel ready, shift your attention to your face. How does it feel now? Focus on the sensations on your face for a while. Notice your eyes, the space between your eyes, your nose, your cheeks, lips, and everything happening there right now.

(Pause for a few seconds)

From there, gradually move your inner gaze down through your neck and upper chest onto your heart. Stay here for a moment. Feel your heart, the space inside and outside it. Sense its movement if you can.

(Pause for a few seconds)

Try now to let your attention rest on your face and heart at the same time.

Can you perceive a connection between these two parts of the body? Perhaps you sense a flow of energy that binds them together; maybe you visualize an image that unites them, or maybe you don't feel anything at all. Whatever experience arises as you hold your attention in that space, allow it to just be. Compassionately study it for a while... Focus on your face and heart. Gather information about yourself in this process.

(Pause for a few seconds)

Your face reaches out to the world, your ears seek sounds of welcome, friendly voices, words of safety.

Your eyes look for cheerful faces, warm smiles, and gestures of peace. Try to feel how your heart responds to this search. Your face and heart are wired for safety and connection. Your face and heart seek co-regulation.

(Pause for a few seconds)

Try to think now how your eyes, the sound of your voice, and your smile open the door to others, sending signals of safety and connection. Try to feel how your heart responds to this invitation to connect. Your face and heart are wired for safety and connection. Your face and heart seek co-regulation.

(Pause for a few seconds)

Now give yourself some time to transition between these two needs of yours... the search for connection, the invitation to connect... Notice what happens to you when you realize that, in the miracle of the encounter, you give and receive co-regulation. Collect information about yourself.

(Pause for a few seconds)

Finally, let go of any focus and give yourself a few moments of open awareness. When you feel fully present, gently open your eyes. Return to the here and now.

After this guided imagery experience, invite participants to share their reflections. Maintain an open, welcoming, and non-judgmental attitude. Some participants may struggle to connect with themselves at such a subtle level. Encourage them lovingly to recognize when they are on the right track. Instill them with confidence that, with practice, their ability to perceive themselves will improve.

4.4 Setting Homework

Regulating Resources Map

This week's homework (taken from Dana, 2018, p. 76) focuses on discovering personal and interpersonal resources that assist in regulating the autonomic nervous system. Follow previous instructions for assigning homework.

Use this map (Figure 4.3) to review activities you can do alone or with others to regulate your nervous system. These resources can help you move up the Autonomic Ladder and return to ventral vagal connection and safety (see Figure 4.4 for a completed example).

Choose one color for the "things I can do on my own" column and another for the "things I can do with others" column.

Start with the survival response you feel most familiar with (sympathetic or dorsal vagal). Ask yourself: "What can I do on my own to get out of here? What can I do with others to get out of here?"

Then, continue with the next row, answering the same questions.

Fill out the ventral vagal section last, this time asking yourself: "What can I do on my own to stay here? What can I do with others to stay here?"

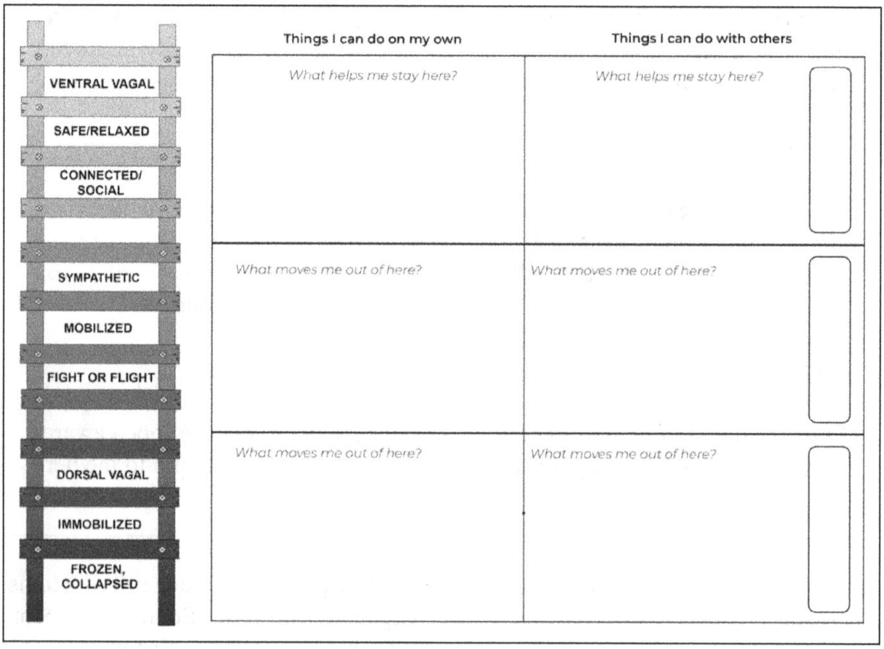

Figure 4.3 Map of Regulating Resources.

From *The Polyvagal Theory in Therapy: Engaging the Rhythm of Regulation* by Deb Dana. Copyright © 2018 by Deb Dana. Used by permission of W. W. Norton & Company, Inc.

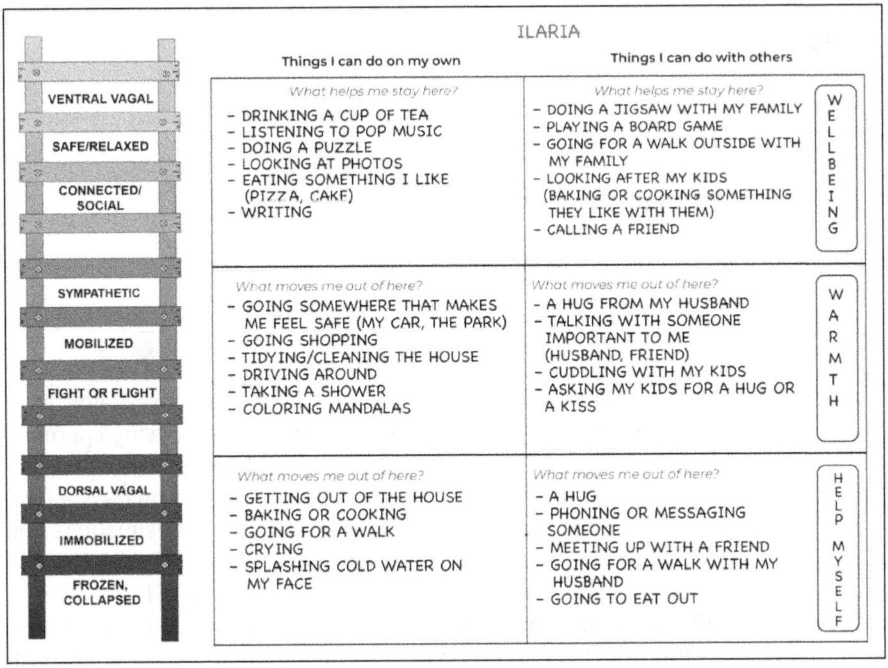

Figure 4.4 An Example Map of Regulating Resources Filled Out by a Course Participant.

4.5 Closing Ritual and Farewell

The group has just concluded the guided imagery activity. For this reason, the closing ritual of the day simply consists of three calming breaths (see the instructions in Session 1).

The meeting ends with you expressing gratitude towards the nervous system of all participants. Encourage them to pay attention to their autonomic responses as often as possible and to use breathing as a key regulatory resource.

The Vagal Brake

The fifth session represents the halfway point in the program. Participants now have a solid understanding of their autonomic world and can describe it using appropriate language. They have begun to establish a connection between their past and present, recognizing that *their autonomic responses do not depend on them but on what happened to them*. They know their triggers and can identify situations that make them feel regulated and connected, having reviewed the set of resources they possess to move out of survival mode and keep themselves balanced. Building on this, today's meeting introduces the concept of the Vagal Brake. Grasping the regulatory function of this biological device will allow the group to master a powerful tool for modulating their autonomic responses and dwelling in a state of optimal activation.

Learning Goals

*   Expanding and enhancing the range of personal and interactive resources for returning to or remaining in a state of autonomic equilibrium through the homework review.
*   Gaining an understanding of the Vagal Brake and experiencing its regulatory function.
*   Understanding that there are new skills to learn to supplement the existing toolkit.

Session Framework

1   Session opening and homework review – 60 minutes
2   Polyvagal Module 5 – 30 minutes
3   Experiential learning: using the Vagal Brake – 50 minutes
4   Setting homework – 10 minutes
5   Closing ritual and farewell – 10 minutes

N.B.: The times indicated are only intended as a guide. The process should be adapted to the group's needs, which we encourage you to prioritize as part of your roadmap.

DOI: 10.4324/9781003560968-10

5.1   Session Opening and Homework Review

After an initial welcome to participants, the instructor briefly summarizes the previous session and leads a discussion of the homework. Invite the group to actively note the resources mentioned by each member. This way, individuals can inspire and enrich each other's skill sets.

5.2   Polyvagal Module 5

Continuing with the theme of regulating resources, the instructor introduces the concept of the *Vagal Brake*, a biological mechanism that helps us maintain a state of balance – or even optimal activation – preventing us from slipping into a sympathetic mobilization response.

What keeps our heartbeat calm and steady under normal circumstances? What speeds it up when we need to perform tasks that require energy or effort? What allows it to return to its regular speed, letting us open up to connection, after going into overdrive due to our survival responses? The answer is the Vagal Brake.

The heart is equipped with a natural pacemaker, called the sinoatrial node. The Vagal Brake is the part of the ventral vagus wired to this biological device. It works just like the brake on a bicycle, ordering our heart muscle to speed up or slow down. Releasing the Vagal Brake activates the sympathetic nervous system. By applying it judiciously, our system controls the amount of incoming energy, maintaining our balance as we run, dance, sunbathe on the lawn, or chat with friends. Operating the Vagal Brake also allows us to return to ventral vagal regulation once we have descended further down the rungs of our Autonomic Ladder into sympathetic activation (Figure 5.1).

The Vagal Brake, therefore, enables us to move flexibly between moments of calm, optimal activation – which lies at the intersection between the ventral vagal and sympathetic – and mobilization (Figure 5.2).

We can all learn strategies to actively engage this biological mechanism, training ourselves to master its use.

5.3   Experiential Learning: Guided Imagery

Using the Vagal Brake

At this point, the group will engage in a classroom activity. Each participant should become aware of possessing a Vagal Brake, and be able to feel, visualize, represent, and/or describe it. Start with a short guided imagery exercise:

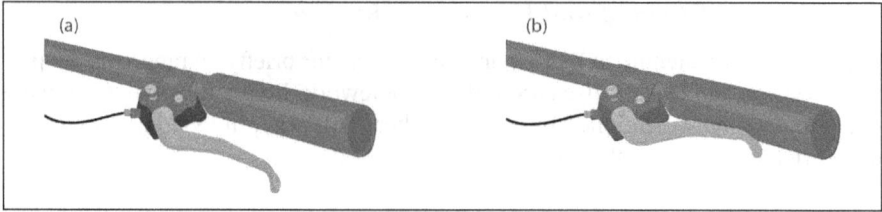

Figure 5.1 (a) and (b) The "Vagal Brake" Acts Like a Bicycle Brake.

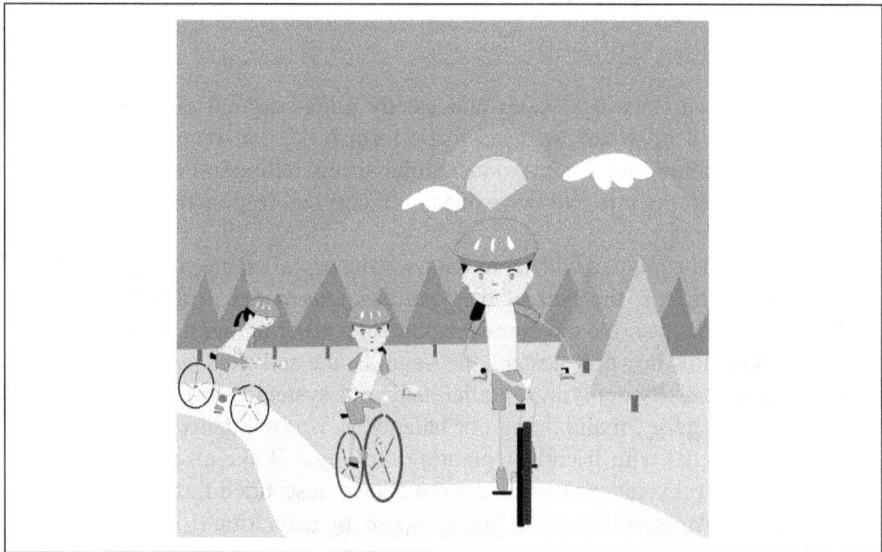

Figure 5.2 The Vagal Brake Enables Us to Move Flexibly through States of Activation and Calm.

Close your eyes gently or, if you wish, let them stay open, gazing softly downward. Allow yourself to be alert and relaxed at the same time. Observe your experience and embrace it as it is. Enter your inner world by focusing on your breathing for a few cycles. Lengthen your breath: inhale and exhale slowly, letting your belly relax.

(Pause for a few seconds)

You know your Shadows. You know what triggers a slight state of mobilization in you. Imagine being in one of those situations. This could be just before delivering a speech in public, or going to an important appointment, or facing a medical exam that is worrying you a little. Visualize yourself in that scenario, whatever resonates for you. Your sympathetic nervous system should be slightly activated, ready for action.

(Pause for a few seconds)

Transport yourself into that situation. Stay there for a while, feel it, mentally recording every detail…

Now actively notice how your heart tends to respond to sympathetic activation. As you let go of your Vagal Brake, your pulse may increase slightly. Remain in that space for a while and observe as your heart prepares to face the challenge…

(Pause for a few seconds)

Now, slow your heart through intentional breathing: inhale for four seconds, pause for two seconds, and exhale for six…

Repeat this breathing pattern five or six times until your heart rate is back to normal and you feel calm.

By breathing this way, you are actively using your Vagal Brake. Gather information about how you perceive your Vagal Brake from within. Note any other physical sensations that emerge through this experience. When you feel ready, gently open your eyes and reconnect to your surroundings.

Through this experience, participants can grasp the essence of the Vagal Brake concept. Now give them the following instructions (Dana, 2020, p. 277):

- Starting from the experience you have just had, consider how you could visualize your Vagal Brake. Which images best represent its regulatory function for you?
- Once you've identified your image, draw it and write down its story in a few words, explaining why you chose it.
- Associate your image of the Vagal Brake with movement and breathing. Remember that when you inhale, you release the brake, increasing your energy. When you exhale, you apply the brake, slowing your energy intake.
- Practice for a few minutes with the movement and breathing you have identified.

Allow 20 minutes for individual work on identifying an image to represent the Vagal Brake, depicting it, and associating it with a movement. Then, divide participants into small groups of three or four for a 30-minute activity. If you conduct the program online, assign them to virtual breakout rooms. Each group member should present their idea of the Vagal Brake to their classmates. Remind everyone to approach each other's contributions with openness and curiosity, avoiding negative comments.

After participants have finished sharing, gather all together and do a quick check to verify that everyone has identified their image.

5.4   Setting Homework

Your Vagal Brake

The homework of the week builds on the activity the group has just completed. Provide participants with the following instructions (see Figure 5.3 for an example of a completed diary).

- Think about your Vagal Brake – your association of image, movement, and breathing.
- Finish or refine your drawing: what does your own personal Vagal Brake look like to you?
- Introduce your Vagal Brake into your daily life, and use it as a resource for regulation.

Fill in your Vagal Brake Diary: When did you use it? Were you in sympathetic activation? How did you respond?

BIANCA			
Time & date	What was happening	What you were feeling (state)	How you used the vagal brake
Mar 3 10:00	I didn't have much time to let my work know whether I would take on new responsibilities	Anxious (sympathetic)	I went for a walk, remembering to breath slowly and deeply.
Mar 5 9:00	A weekend away with my friends was called off	Depressed (dorso vagal)	I cleaned my house from top to bottom. The sense of shutting down I experienced before was replaced by anger. At that point, I began to focus on my breathing and making longer exhales, as I had learned, which helped calm me down.
Mar 14 9:00	For work I have to quickly learn to speak Spanish	Anxious (sympathetic)	When the anxiety came on, I put my hand on my heart and relaxed my muscles. I felt my heart beating more slowly.

Figure 5.3 The Vagal Brake: An Example of a Table Filled Out by a Participant for Homework.

5.5 Closing Ritual and Farewell

Turn Your Head and Breathe

The closing exercise of the day consists of three rotations of the head – first clockwise and then counterclockwise – accompanied by intentional breathing. Invite participants to do the following (Figure 5.4).

- Position your head so that your gaze points forward.
- Turn your chin towards your left shoulder. As you breathe in, lean your head back and slowly roll it towards your right shoulder.
- As you breathe out, turn your head from the right shoulder towards your breastbone and then towards your left shoulder. If it helps, visualize a marble (your head) rotating around a central point (your neck) to make a circle. Repeat the movement two more times. If leaning your head back is painful, simply turn it forwards, making half a circle.
- Repeat the entire sequence but in reverse, from the right shoulder back to the left.

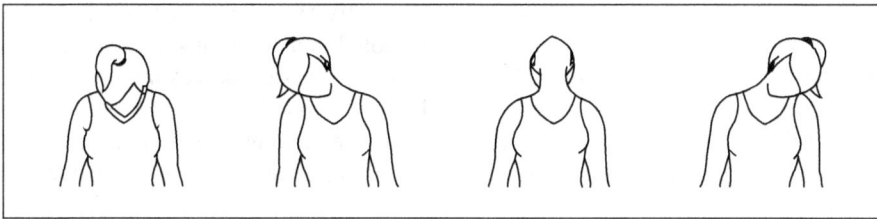

Figure 5.4 Turn Your Head and Breathe.

At the end of the experience, invite the participants to turn their attention inward and note the sensations generated by the exercise. Wrap up the meeting by thanking the nervous system of all participants. Encourage them to be mindful of their autonomic responses as often as possible and to use their Vagal Brake as a daily regulatory resource.

Breathwork

In the first half of their journey, the group has acquired a series of tools – like maps – for recognizing their habitual autonomic responses, the neuroception that triggers certain states, and what brings them back into regulation. They have begun to view their own physiology with compassion, gaining insight into its innate intelligence from within. They have started to savor the experience of co-regulation with you and each other. From this point onward, participants learn to take the reins as "drivers" of their nervous systems, modulating their activation. It is time to create a new "springboard" for themselves, a foundation rooted in a sense of security and connection from which to explore the world. Today's session delves into one of the most effective means of building this new biological platform: breathwork.

This meeting marks the beginning of the highly experiential part of the program, focusing on breathing, sound, and movement. This learning phase is extensive and requires your direct involvement. However, you do not need any special skills to conduct these sessions. Anyone can do it. You don't have to be a great singer, a yoga master, or an expert in anything else. As an instructor, you only need to experiment and reflect on the exercises beforehand. Ensure you are familiar with the activities before introducing them to the group. Practice will allow you to master them and appreciate their immense benefits.

Learning Goals

- Expanding knowledge of the Vagal Brake through the homework review and others' experiences, broadening the range of applicable situations.
- Understanding that breathwork is a powerful tool for regulating the autonomic nervous system.
- Experimenting with various breathing techniques.

Session Framework

1. Session opening and homework review – 60 minutes
2. Polyvagal Module 6 – 10 minutes
3. Experiential learning – 60 minutes
4. Setting homework – 10 minutes
5. Closing ritual and farewell – 10 minutes

DOI: 10.4324/9781003560968-11

N.B.: The times indicated are only intended as a guide. The process should be adapted to the group's needs, which we encourage you to prioritize as part of your roadmap.

6.1   Session Opening and Homework Review

After an initial welcome, briefly recap the previous session and read through the homework. Invite the group to take note of the various situations in which other participants have integrated the Vagal Brake into their lives.

6.2   Polyvagal Module 6

Let the group know that they have reached the halfway point in the program, a milestone worth celebrating. This marks the beginning of a new phase, in which participants will learn several simple and easy-to-apply tools for writing a new narrative for themselves. The goal is to stop being held hostage by one's own neuroception, and instead to become the screenwriter, director, and lead actor of a new plot. Introduce the theme of the day: breathwork (Figure 6.1). You can use the following example script.

> Breathing is an immediate "switch" for our autonomic nervous system, helping us regulate our physical and emotional states.
>
> Just as no two moments are alike, no two breaths are alike. Breathing is the tangible sign that we are alive, here and now, a miraculous action that marks the beginning and end of our existence.
>
> We often forget to notice our breathing, letting it occur in the background. Yet, if you think about it, the number of biological processes involved when we inhale and exhale is astounding. On average, adults take between 12 and 18 breaths per minute, which amounts to about 20,160 a day – an impressive number.
>
> Well, each of these breaths carries a promise: the potential for transformation. Change begins with becoming aware of our breath. However, noticing it means also venturing into our mind space, as breathing and mental activity are, in fact, intimately linked. They are closely intertwined. For some, merely noticing the breath immediately has a calming and centering effect. For others, focusing on breathing can sound an alarm. Through neuroception, our breath often serves as the gateway to our deepest, sometimes painful emotions.
>
> Each breath also allows us to guide our bodies towards safety and connection. But for this to happen, we must become like explorers. We must be willing to experiment with new and intentional ways of breathing with curiosity and an open mind.

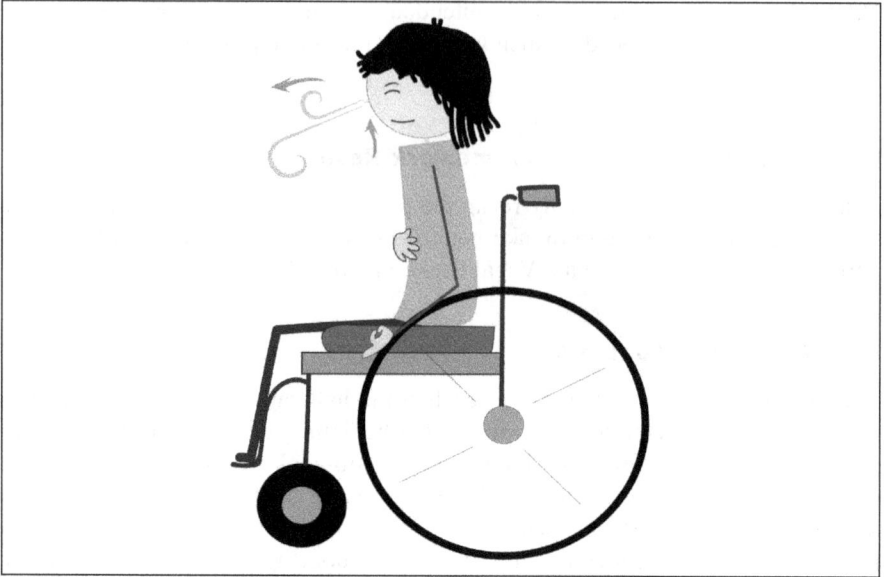

Figure 6.1 With Every Breath We Have an Opportunity to Change.

6.3 *Experiential Learning: Breathwork*

Before diving into the exercises below, set up the workspace. If the program is conducted in person, prepare the room with yoga mats and – if you like – meditation cushions or benches. If the program is delivered online, invite participants to have this material ready and ensure they position their webcam so that you can see them doing the activities.

We have recommended several exercises for this module, but it isn't necessary to cover them all. Choose the ones that best suit your group size and characteristics, your personal sensibilities, and the time available. You might consider scheduling an extra session to do some of these activities. This will give you time to get through them without rushing and enable you to monitor the participants closely. It is advisable to mix in moments for sharing group experiences, as recommended in Chapter 3.

As emphasized earlier, it is crucial that you have tried the activities you select and lead them with ease and naturalness. Don't simply tell the participants what to do. Engage with the exercises alongside them. Your example will motivate them. Moreover, you will offer your nervous system in service of the group's sense of safety and connection.

In yoga, breathing exercises are called *pranayama*. They are used to modulate our *prana*, our vital energy. As such, they are essential tools for physical, mental, and spiritual well-being. These age-old practices inspire some of the breathing techniques presented here.

Before experimenting with breathwork, it is essential first to find your breath within your body, recognize it, and follow where it leads. The first three exercises aim to help participants develop this level of awareness, so they can consciously use their breath as a switch for ventral vagal regulation. You might introduce this section of the program with an opening message like this:

Since our first meeting, we have been honing our ability to observe our breathing. We have seen how slow, deep breaths soothe our autonomic nervous system. Now, we are going to explore a long series of breathing techniques together.

The first step is to perform the exercises correctly. You will gradually become familiar with them, especially as you practice at home. Try not to be hard on yourself. Learning takes time. As you continue, you will be able to identify the breathing techniques that are most beneficial for you and your nervous system. You can then apply these techniques to enhance your daily life.

Exercise 1 – Feel Your Breath

•   Sit, stand, or lie on your back, whichever is most comfortable. Relax and turn your attention inward. If it helps, close your eyes or gently lower your gaze (Figure 6.2).

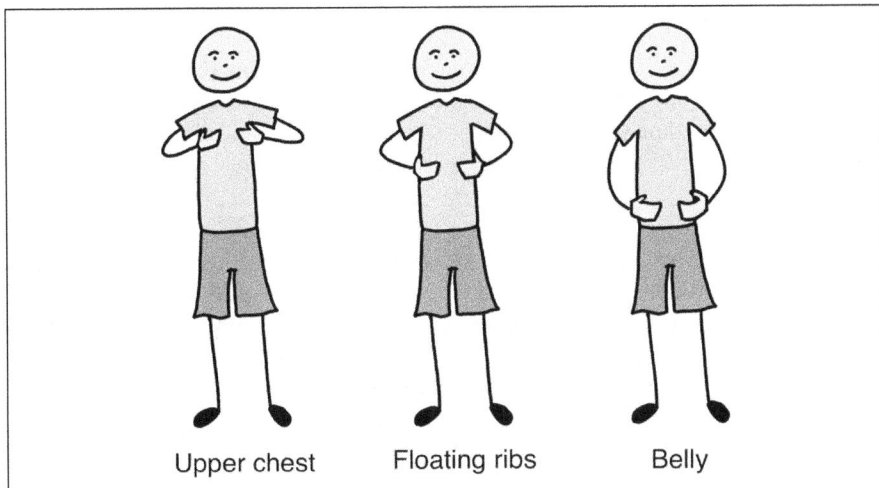

Upper chest   Floating ribs   Belly

Figure 6.2 "Feel Your Breath".

- Place your hands on the upper part of your chest, slightly apart. As you breathe in and out, notice the natural movements occurring in your chest. Feel all the sensations.
- Now, move your hands to the sides of your torso and gently hug your lower ribs. As you inhale and exhale, pay attention to the movements in this area. Savor all the sensations.
- Finally, place your hands on your belly. Inhale and exhale while observing the movement in your abdomen as you breathe. Notice what you feel inside.

The activity should take about five minutes in total.

Exercise 2 – Slow Breathing

- Stay in the position from Exercise 1. Imagine you have a pot with murky water at the bottom. To have clean water, what do you do first? Empty out the pot to remove the sediment. Do the same with your lungs: breathe out deeply to clear them before making space for fresh air.
- Breathe out slowly, emptying yourself completely. Then breathe in.
- Breathe steadily in and out, aiming for each exhale and inhale to last four seconds.

This exercise should take about three minutes. Conclude by encouraging the group to notice the effects of this slow, regular breathing on their mind-body system.

Exercise 3 – On Your Belly

Breathing while lying on our stomach makes us aware of how the abdomen moves with each breath (Figure 6.3). This position helps us connect with how our natural breathing rhythm feels. Guide participants through the following exercise for about five minutes. Remember to ask them to share any effects they notice afterward.

- Lie on your stomach on the mat with your hands beneath your forehead. If it is more comfortable, you can make fists with your hands or use a yoga block. Place a cushion under your hips if you feel discomfort in your lower back.
- Inhale and exhale naturally, without forcing it. Notice through contact with the mat how your breath moves in your body. Follow its sensations, breath by breath, as it makes its journey through your nostrils, down your throat, into your chest, and finally into your belly.

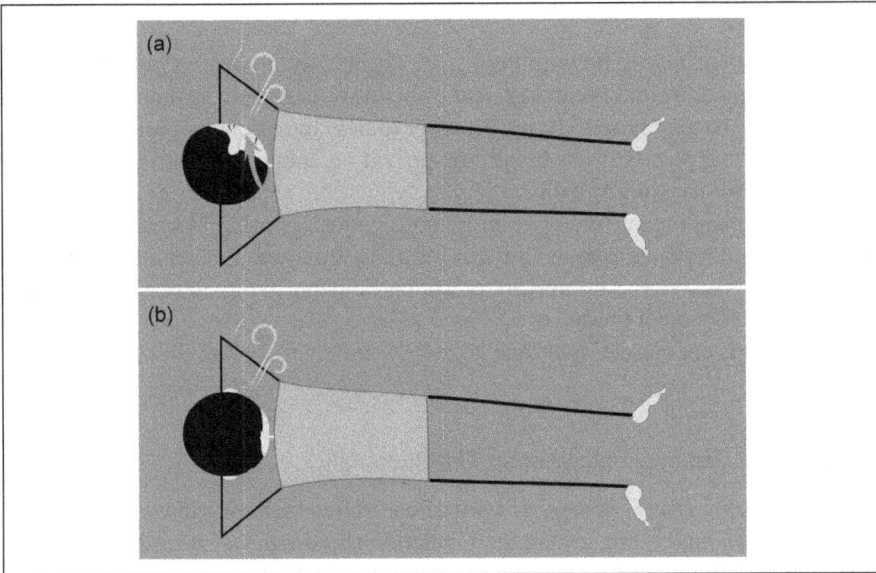

Figure 6.3 (a) and (b) "On Your Belly".

Exercise 4 – A Sigh of Relief

We might not always notice when we sigh, but we do it more often than we think. Sighing can express a variety of emotions – from relief and contentment to sadness and anxiety. And let's not forget the sighs of love!

Our physiology has endowed us with this instant, automatic behavior, allowing us to return to balance from activation. Sighing can feel like letting go of a heavy burden. With each sigh, we improve our state and guide ourselves towards lightness and tranquility.

Sighing can be a regulatory resource (Dana, 2018, p. 136), and we can learn to produce sighs intentionally through the following exercise:

- Sit or stand comfortably with your back upright but relaxed. Close your eyes or soften your gaze.
- Breathe in through your nose, counting to four.
- Hold your breath for two seconds.
- Breathe out for six seconds, controlling the airflow. Maintain your posture as you let out a loud sigh. You should feel a gentle vibration in your throat.
- Spend two or three minutes in this space. How did this type of breathing affect you?

Exercise 5 – Blowing Bubbles

What do bubbles have to do with Polyvagal Theory? Well, making soap bubbles is an exercise in controlled breathing. Not only do we learn to coordinate our mouth muscles, but we also practice long, steady exhales. Intentionally creating bubbles helps us become aware of our breathing, providing another fun and effective way to modulate our nervous system.

If you are leading the exercise in person, gather soap bubble wands for each participant and let them play with them for a few minutes. If teaching online, you can assign this activity as homework or ask participants to purchase a bubble wand beforehand and have it ready.

At the end, encourage everyone to take a moment to feel the effects of the exercise.

Exercise 6 – Geometric Breathing: The Rectangle

"Rectangular breathing" is another form of controlled breathing in which the exhalation is intentionally longer than the inhalation (Figure 6.4). Like other breathing exercises, it can help us regulate our autonomic state. Here are the steps:

- Visualize a rectangle with long sides twice as long as the short ones. Trace it in the air with your finger.
- Now trace the rectangle with your breath, breathing in on the short sides and out on the long sides. Draw the first short side, inhaling for two seconds, then the first long side, exhaling for four seconds. Continue to trace the rectangle, breathing through the third and fourth sides in the same way.
- Do this for two or three minutes. What impact did this type of breathing have on your body and mind?

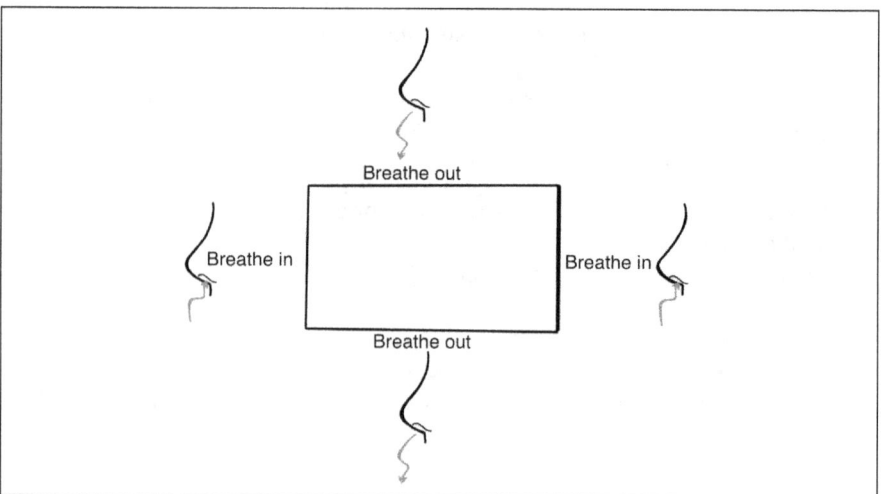

Figure 6.4 "Geometric Breathing": The Rectangle.

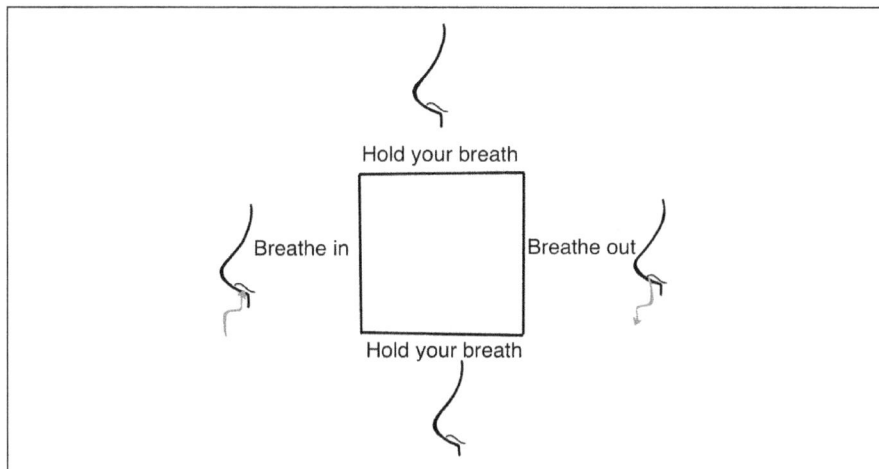

Figure 6.5 "Geometric Breathing": The Square.

Exercise 7 – Geometric Breathing: The Square

An image of a square can also help control breathing. In this case the inhalations and exhalations are the same length (Figure 6.5).

- Imagine a square for this exercise. Each side corresponds to an action: inhale, hold your breath, exhale, hold, and so on.
- Breathe in for a mental count of four (side 1).
- Hold your breath for four seconds (side 2).
- Breathe out for a mental count of four (side 3).
- Hold your breath for four seconds (side 4).

Encourage participants to practice geometric breathing at home. As they become more experienced, they can experiment with different shapes, gradually enlarging their squares or rectangles. As the length of their sides increases, so does the length of their breaths in and out, to five, six, seven seconds, etc.

Exercise 8 – The Breath of Joy

This exercise is a compassionate invitation to climb the Autonomic Ladder and enter a ventral vagal state. Combining breath with movement stimulates the vagus nerve very effectively, as we will see in Session 8. In addition, the intention to open up to joy aims to help participants anchor on to positive emotions. As you guide the group through the activity, instruct them to breathe joy in and breathe joy out, allowing the musicality of your voice to act as a strong co-regulating force. Before performing the exercise as a whole, it's advisable to demonstrate the movements one by one using these instructions:

- Sit or stand upright, with your feet facing forward, a hip-width apart. Keep your back straight and relaxed, shoulders soft, not up to your ears. Clasp your hands in front of your chest, with your index fingers pointing up towards your chin.
- Interlace your fingers as you breathe in, imagining that you are inhaling joy, filling your lungs with it like a delicious scent.
- Stretch your arms out in front of you, keeping your hands intertwined, palms outward, as you release the air and imagine yourself *breathing out joy*.
- Raise your arms level with your ears, keeping your hands intertwined with your palms facing the ceiling. Take in the air and imagine *breathing in joy*.
- Separate your hands and slowly bring your arms down by your sides as you release the air and imagine yourself *breathing out joy*.
- Bring your arms behind your back and clasp your hands while you take in the air and imagine *breathing in joy*.
- Bring your arms back to the starting position, with your hands clasped in front of your chest, while releasing the air and imagining yourself *breathing out joy*.

Once the group has mastered the sequence, lead them through the entire exercise, demonstrating the movements while saying, "Breathe in joy" and "Breathe out joy". Invite them to join you in mentally repeating the phrases. The activity should last about six to eight minutes. At the end, invite participants to reflect on the effect of the exercise on their mind–body connection.

Exercise 9 – Ujjayi, or The Ocean Within Us

Ujjayi is a breathing practice used to calm the mind, relax the body, and enhance awareness of our breath. It consists of slow, deep breaths through the nose, with a slight throat contraction, which creates a sound similar to ocean waves. It helps slow down the breathing rate, increases oxygenation, and promotes focus and concentration.

Ujjayi can be done standing, sitting, or lying down (Figure 6.6). It is a very fluid breath, with both inhales and exhales lasting about 4 seconds. However, before practicing Ujjayi, you need to find it, as follows:

- First inhale through your mouth while partially closing your throat.
- Now, exhale as if you are fogging up a glass in front of you. You should produce a hoarse sound, a kind of hiss.
- Next, while keeping your mouth open, try inhaling, producing the same sound in the back of your throat.

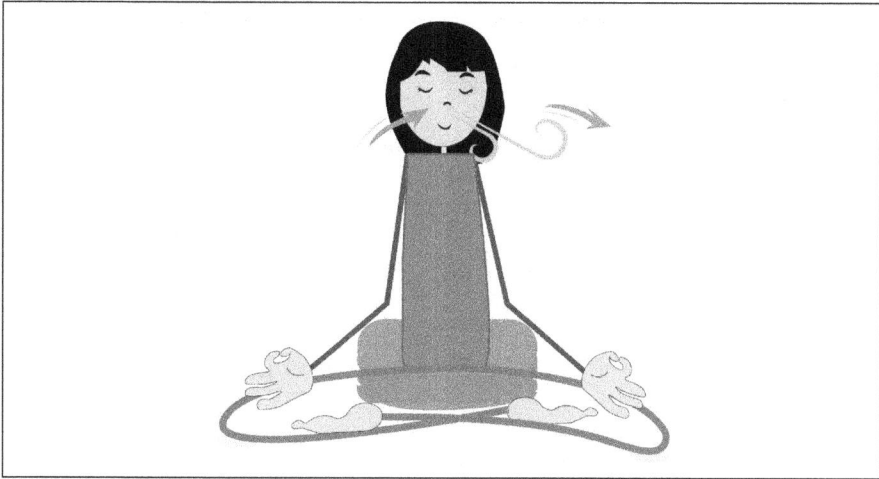

Figure 6.6 "The Ocean Within Us": Ujjayi.

- Once you find the right throat position and sound, practice it with your mouth closed. Start by producing sound only as you exhale. When you begin to feel comfortable with the technique, add sound to the inhale too.
- Practice for a couple of minutes. At the end of the activity, take a few moments to reflect on its impact on your body and mind.

Exercise 10 – Kapalabhati, or Breath of Fire

Kapalabhati is a breathing technique used to cleanse the mind and body, increase energy, and sharpen concentration. It helps us get rid of carbon dioxide and take in oxygen. From a polyvagal perspective, it is an exceptional tool for pulling the autonomic nervous system out of dorsal vagal shutdown. It involves rhythmic exhalations through the nose, supported by the movement of the abdominal muscles, followed by passive inhalation. *Note: this exercise is contraindicated for people suffering from hypertension, heart disease, inguinal hernia, epilepsy, dizziness, glaucoma, frequent nosebleeds, or those with a history of stroke.*

- Blow your nose well and keep a tissue handy.
- Sit comfortably with your back straight, your abdomen relaxed, and your hands resting on your knees. Close your eyes.
- Imagine you have a fly buzzing around the tip of your nose, and you want to drive it away.
- Take in air through your nostrils, then emit a short, vigorous breath out through your nose, as if you want to blow away the fly. Use your upper abdominal muscles to breathe out.

- Now repeat the exercise, keeping your back straight as best you can. Breathe in and out through your nose this way for ten breaths.
- At the end of the cycle, relax into a natural, passive breath.

Kapalabhati is usually practiced for three cycles of ten consecutive breaths. Since it is a high-impact breathing technique, we suggest starting with a single cycle. At the end, encourage the group to gather for a few moments and note how they feel.

Exercise 11 – Bhramari, or Bee Breathing

Bhramari is a type of noisy breathing. The inhalation is followed by a closed-mouth exhale, producing a buzzing sound like a bee. The resulting vibration helps to relieve tension and stress. Allow your participants to experience its benefits, by guiding them through the following exercise:

- Sit comfortably with your back straight and your hands resting on your knees. Close your eyes and relax your whole body.
- Inhale slowly, without filling your lungs completely. Exhale with softly closed lips and relaxed jaw, making a buzzing sound like a bee. If you think it would help, put your index fingers in your ears or gently cover your ears with your hands so that you can hear the sound better.
- Continue until your lungs are empty.
- Repeat the cycle for three to four minutes. With this type of *pranayama*, note that the exhalation naturally tends to lengthen.

Conclude by inviting participants to reflect on this exercise's impact on their mind–body connection.

Exercise 12 – Sitali, the Cooling Breath

This *pranayama* is used to cool the body. It involves a specific tongue position, so allow time for experimentation until participants master it. This technique can be used in hot weather, after a workout, or during moments of anger to let off emotional steam. It's an excellent resource for calming down, especially before bed. Here is how to do it (Figure 6.7):

- Sit comfortably with your back straight and your hands resting on your knees. Close your eyes and relax your whole body.
- First, experiment with your tongue. Can you roll it up like a straw? If not, don't worry: whether or not we can do this depends on our genes. Open your mouth and stick your tongue out. If you can, roll it into a straw shape. If not,

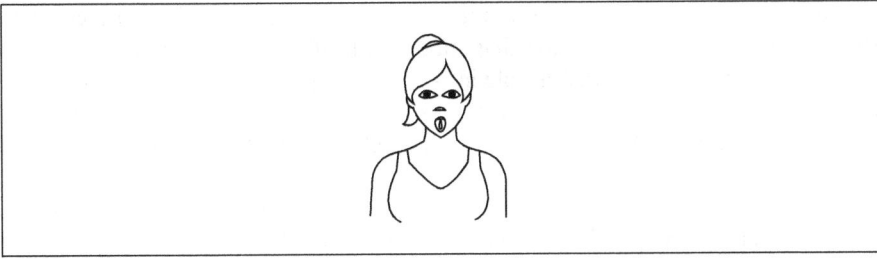

Figure 6.7 Sitali: Tongue Position.

place it between your lips or gently push it against the teeth, on the floor of your mouth. Explore positions until you find the one that works best for you.

- Once your tongue is in place, inhale as if you are sipping air through a straw. Fill your lungs for four seconds while imagining you're cleansing your tongue with your breath. Your shoulders should remain low and relaxed without rising towards your ears. Focus on the sound you make as you breathe in. It is a healing sound.
- Now close your mouth and hold your breath for a few seconds. If it feels comfortable, rest your chin on your breastbone; otherwise, keep it up, looking in front of you. If you have laid your head down, lift it up and slowly exhale through your nose for six seconds. Slow down your breathing as much as possible.

Repeat the cycle five times, and afterward, encourage the group to reflect on the sensations this exercise leaves behind.

Exercise 13 – Diaphragmatic Breathing

Let's start with some theory, as understanding our anatomy can help us get the most from this exercise. We breathe into and out of our lungs, which are contained within the rib cage. The main respiratory muscle is the diaphragm: this has a characteristic dome shape and divides the chest cavity from the abdominal cavity. When we inhale, the diaphragm contracts and lowers; during exhalation, it returns to its original position. As it lowers, it makes room for the lungs to expand and draw air into the airways.

During breathing, the chest cavity expands and contracts as a result of two distinct mechanisms:

- contraction of the diaphragm, which moves downwards and upwards;
- contraction of the chest muscles.

Breathing is a synergy between these two actions. Why, then, differentiate between *thoracic* and *diaphragmatic breathing*? Thoracic breathing focuses on the action of the chest and neck muscles, while diaphragmatic breathing gives the diaphragm a workout.

Our lives are filled with stressors that cause us anxiety. We live in a constant state of alarm, which makes the diaphragm stiff, affecting its function. The diaphragm is the most *emotional* muscle in our body: it gets tense when we experience life events, sorrows, and difficulties, but also hunched posture, computer work, and a sedentary lifestyle. We need to regain the ability to breathe, getting the best out of this extraordinary muscle.

Diaphragmatic, or abdominal, breathing refers to a type of breathing in which the diaphragm allows maximum lung expansion. Therefore, air can penetrate deep down and to the sides, filling every corner of your lungs. Diaphragmatic breathing calms us, makes us feel more alive, and improves digestion. Deep, with a long, slow exhale, this technique is key to stimulating the vagus nerve, slowing heart rate, and lowering blood pressure.

Babies are born breathing this way. As we grow up, we unlearn, but it's never too late to reclaim this skill, savoring all its regulatory and regenerative effects. The optimal position for diaphragmatic breathing is lying down, with your knees bent and your feet firmly planted on the ground. If lying down isn't an option, you can still practice the exercise sitting upright. Find the position that suits you best.

- Close your eyes and relax your body.
- Place your hands on your chest, breathing naturally through your nose. Try to feel your breath under your fingers. Notice how your chest rises with each inhale and lowers with each exhale. The sensation may be subtle at first but, with time, you will become more aware of how the breath moves in this part of your body. Take your time: you are getting in touch with your chest breath.
- Next, move your hands to your abdomen. Try to breathe through your nose, producing longer and deeper inhalations and exhalations. You should feel your abdomen rising under your hands. This doesn't mean you're breathing with your belly; it's simply your diaphragm contracting and moving your bowels down. Practice this long, deep breathing for a while. You are on the path to diaphragmatic breathing.
- Finally, place one hand in the center of the chest and the other on your belly. Breathe in and out through your nose. Without tensing up, try to keep your upper chest still while the air moves downwards, filling up your lungs. Breathe with your diaphragm alone. You will know you are doing it correctly when your chest barely moves and your belly inflates and deflates as if there were a balloon inside. Try to keep your shoulders still and soft. Focus on the length and depth of your breath.

This activity should last about 10 minutes. At the end, invite participants to regroup and share how the exercise has impacted their physical and emotional state.

ELISA

What breaths can I use to bring my autonomic state back into a regulated condition?

1) BEE BREATHING

I love it. I do it with my daughter as well. It's both a game and a way to co-regulate. We have fun and feel connected at the same time.

2) THE BREATH OF JOY

This breath has improved my mood a lot and I've decided to practice it every morning as soon as I wake up. I think because it is associated with movements of my arms and back, it gives me a lot of relief. On the exhale, I can release all the tension that has been building up in those parts of my body.

3) RECTANGLE BREATHING

I like it, because the longer exhale helps me lower my level of sympathetic activation.

RICHARD

What breaths can I use to bring my autonomic state back into a regulated condition?

The breathing technique that has come to my rescue most easily and most frequently these days is The Breath of Joy. I applied it both as taught and also in a more practical way, in moments when I felt the need, such as while I was involved in an unpleasant argument or while I was driving. Practicing The Breath of Joy in my mind has made it easier for me to calm down and become less aggressive. The second breath that I found pleasant is the Ujjayi. Lengthening the exhalation phase and focusing on the glottis and diaphragm helps me tremendously to decompress and move more easily into the ventral vagal state. In third place is Bee Breathing. It is a pleasant game which helps me by focusing on modulating my breath and making my diaphragm move, and humming is just as calming as a lullaby. It increases my concentration and improves my mental clarity.

Figure 6.8 Breathwork: Examples of Homework Filled Out by Course Participants.

6.4   Setting Homework

Choose Your Breaths

While introducing the homework for the week, follow the guidelines previously provided. Give participants a handout describing the assignment (Figure 6.8 illustrates an example of a homework assignment from a course participant).

Throughout today's session, you have experimented with various breathing techniques. Using the handouts, revisit and practice the exercises we did today in class as often as possible. Your breath is a strong indicator of your autonomic state and can reveal much about your experiences. Observe it with curiosity. Whenever possible, pause and ask yourself:

- How am I breathing right now?
- What Shadow – or Light – prompted me to breathe this way?
- Where am I on my Autonomic Ladder?
- What breathing techniques can I use to regulate my autonomic state?

Experiment and select two or three techniques that feel most effective for you. Use them whenever you have the chance.

Describe three episodes in which you used your breath as a resource, answering the following questions:

- When did you use your breath as a resource?
- Which breathing techniques did you apply?
- Which autonomic state were you in?
- How did you respond?

6.5   Closing Ritual and Farewell

Conclude the meeting by expressing gratitude for the nervous systems of all participants. Encourage them to remain vigilant about their autonomic responses and to use breathing as a daily regulatory resource.

Session 7

Sound

The highly experiential section of the program continues this meeting. In the previous session, participants engaged in a learning model largely centered on hands-on activities as a pathway to deeper cognitive understanding. They experimented using breathwork as a way to actively modulate their autonomic states and are beginning to apply their newfound polyvagal skills in everyday life. Today, the focus is on sound. In addition to being a powerful vehicle for conveying signals of safety or danger, sound is an extraordinary tool for stimulating the vagus nerve. The session will explore both of these aspects.

Learning Goals

- Consolidating the idea that breathing can serve as a resource for autonomic regulation, and broadening the range of situations in which this is applicable through others' examples.
- Understanding the importance of sound as a major vehicle for transmitting safety or danger signals, a catalyst for autonomic responses, and a tool for stimulating and toning up the vagus nerve.
- Experiencing a range of sound-focused activities.

Session Framework

1. Session opening and homework review – 60 minutes
2. Polyvagal Module 7 – 30 minutes
3. Experiential learning – 60 minutes
4. Setting homework – 10 minutes
5. Closing ritual and farewell – 5 minutes

N.B.: The times indicated are only intended as a guide. The process should be adapted to the group's needs, which we encourage you to prioritize as part of your roadmap.

DOI: 10.4324/9781003560968-12

7.1 Session Opening and Homework Review

After a warm welcome, the instructor briefly summarizes the previous session and proceeds to discuss the completed homework assignments. Invite the group to actively note the various situations in which their peers have used breathing as a regulating resource in their daily lives.

7.2 Polyvagal Module 7

Across all cultures, sound is used to bring people together. From folk songs to religious ceremonies, activities like singing, humming, and chanting have always been vital collective experiences. Since the dawn of time, people have recited fairy tales or nursery rhymes and sung lullabies to soothe children. They read poems to declare their love or despair, or whistle when they are happy. Sound production signals to others how we feel and is an implicit invitation to join in.

Using the voice purposefully has very real benefits for our overall well-being. If we look at this human behavior through the polyvagal lens, chanting, humming, and singing promote proper breathing, stimulate our vagus nerve, and facilitate co-regulation when practiced with others.

Introduce today's theme with a brief theoretical introduction on the strong connection between sound and neuroception. You may find the following script helpful:

Each day, our bodies receive thousands of different sound stimuli. From the alarm clock in the morning to the noise around our home, the traffic on our way to work, the voices of those we interact with, and the rustling of leaves paired with the chirping of birds while walking in the park, we are constantly bombarded by sound. Often, we are not even aware that we are *listening*, and have even less awareness of the impact of these sounds on our nervous system. Yet, sound is an incredibly powerful cue for our neuroception, capable of bringing light into our life or evoking a shadow (see the Map of Lights and Shadows in Session 3). It often triggers a specific autonomic response, even before we can see the source of safety or danger we may have to face. It is like when a fire breaks out. We are likely to hear and understand the significance of the siren before we can see the flames.

But why are we so sensitive to sound?

Well, the answer lies in our evolution. Back in the mists of time, individuals who could detect the sound of a predator approaching before seeing it had a greater chance of survival. This allowed them to monitor their environment without directly confronting threats, refining their fight-or-flight response over generations to be incredibly quick and effective. Today we no longer live in the wild. The luckiest among us lead sheltered lives, not forced to engage in a daily struggle for survival. But our biology remains essentially the same, with our nervous system still reacting to this type of primal alarm. We carry this ancestral imprint within us. Consequently, our neuroception still translates high-frequency sounds as warning signals, bringing out instincts of care and protection in us. For example, a baby crying prompts a physical reaction before we form the thought: "My child may be in danger".

Low, deep frequencies, on the other hand, remind our bodies of the terrifying roar of a large animal chasing us, prompting our bodies to prepare to attack or flee.

Let us now move on from the evolution of our species and focus on the miracle of a human infant's development inside their mother's womb. Together with touch, hearing is among the first senses we develop. But what exactly do we hear? What vibrations reach us? We pick up noises from the surrounding environment, muffled by the amniotic fluid. Yet, the most frequent and intense sounds are those generated by our mother. Through her voice and heartbeat, the child growing inside her forges a bond with her. At this stage of life, we could say that "mom" is experienced mostly through sound. Once born, the baby cannot see further than three feet away. Their mother's voice – the sound, rhythm, and cadence – is essential for conveying reassurance and a sense of safety ("I can hear my mom nearby; therefore, I must be safe" (Figure 7.1)). Thus, sound shapes our neuroception, even before we can see the world around us. From a very early age, our nervous system learns to react to sound stimuli through specific pathways controlled by the vagus nerve.

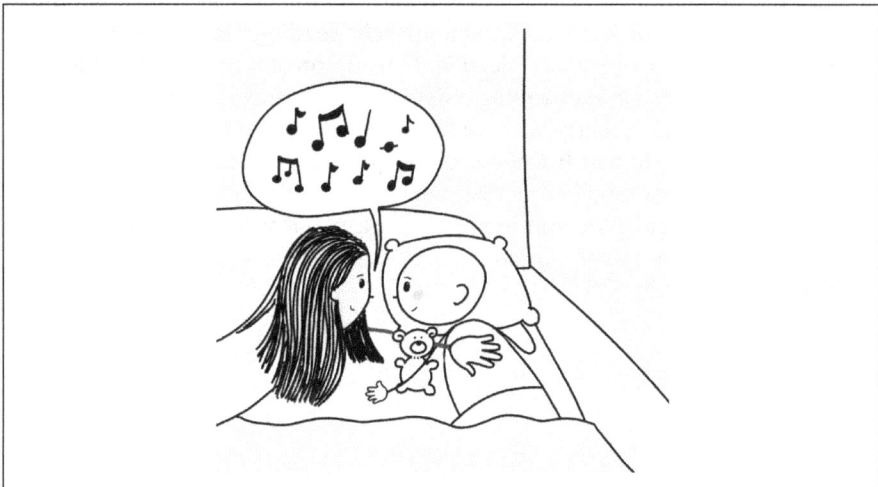

Figure 7.1 A Mother's Voice: One of the Main Safety Signals for a Newborn.

At this point, introduce the idea that even among adults the sound of the human voice conveys signals of safety or danger. The way people talk to each other sends subtle yet powerful cues, representing an invitation or an obstacle to connection. How we speak is a nuanced channel of communication between the nervous systems involved (Figure 7.2).

Seeing signs of security in others – a smile, a certain type of look, a nod of the head – and hearing it in their voice go hand in hand. Early on, the baby's nervous system identifies their mother's voice as one of their primary safety signals and resources for regulation. From that moment on, throughout our lives, we are neurologically wired to detect underlying messages, beyond mere words, from the people we interact with. Are they trustworthy or should we keep our distance? Our neuroception bases this assessment on a series of factors – the rhythm, frequency, duration, and intensity of speech – more than the content itself. Prosody, that is, the voice's musicality (or lack of it) is key. A droning, monotonous voice, or one pitched too high or loud, triggers a danger alarm. On the flip side, a well-modulated voice with a harmonious timbre and rhythm serves as an invitation to connect. Think of the word "attunement". When we are "in tune" with another person we share the same frequency and wavelength. The sound of our voices produces harmony, our neuroception signals its approval, and co-regulation can take place.

Before we explore how sound affects our bodies, let us pause to consider the intimate link between our breath and our voice. Short, shallow breathing results in hurried, broken speech, sending warning signals to those around us. Conversely, deep and steady breathing leads to relaxed and measured speech, conveying safety. In short, our habitual breathing patterns, and consequently how we speak, reflect our autonomic world. In fight-or-flight mode, our breath becomes quicker, our voice is higher, and our speech accelerates. In contrast, when we dwell in the warm embrace of the ventral vagal state, our breathing is easy, our voice flows in a lower tone, and we can savor the sound, sense, and meaning of every word uttered.

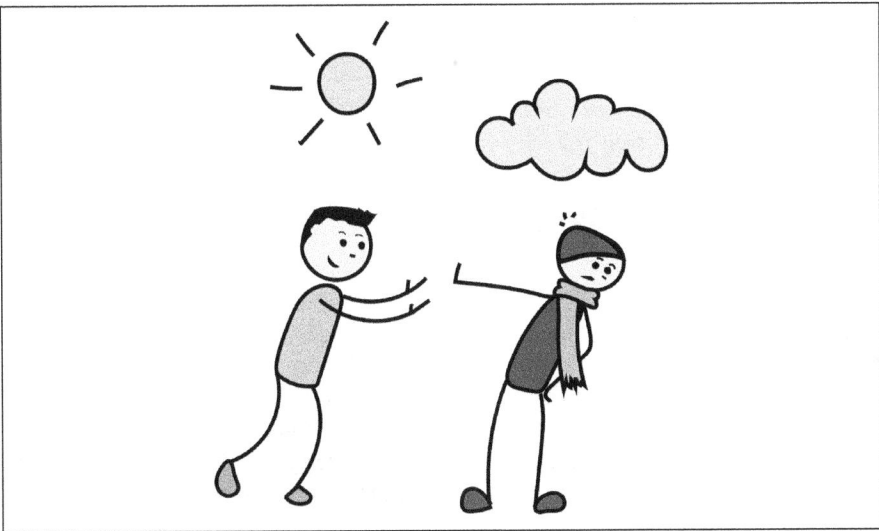

7.2 *Safety* and Danger in Relationships

7.3   *Experiential Learning: Experimenting with Sound*

The experiential learning segment consists of three sections, each featuring a specific type of activity. The first part focuses on sound production. You will guide the group in using their voices as a tool for regulating the vagus nerve. The second section explores prosody (stress and intonation) and investigates its effects on several levels. The third and final part centers on listening, exploring how incoming sounds impact the autonomic nervous system. Sounds can both stimulate our neuroceptive danger responses and serve as an anchor that brings us back into safety, and ventral vagal connection.

Before starting, set up the workspace. If the program is being conducted in person, prepare the room with chairs, meditation cushions, or benches. For the listening activities, provide a fairly powerful speaker. You can play the tracks directly from your computer if you are teaching online. There are audio tracks available from the online resources for this book for all exercises marked with an asterisk (*). For the exercises involving using the voice, be aware that videoconferencing platforms, due to an issue with sound delay, make it difficult for participants to talk or sing in sync and hear each other clearly. Some voices might be audible, while others get lost in the background. Above all, the choir effect is impossible to achieve. Therefore, when inviting participants to perform these exercises, you have two options: either tolerate the din or ask everyone to mute their microphone while singing, humming, or chanting.

Below is a set of recommended activities for this module. Choose the ones appropriate for your teaching style, group size, and available time. As with the previous module, consider spreading this session over two meetings to allow for more in-depth engagement with the various exercises. Incorporate moments for participants to share their experiences, as highlighted in Chapter 3. Keep in mind that working with one's voice can be a very intimate and sensitive experience. Receive the sounds of your participants like a gift. In this segment, more than others, it is crucial to create a safe and welcoming environment in which judgment is suspended. Finally, be mindful to keep your nervous system aligned with the group's needs.

Exercise 1 – Making Sounds: Vowels*

The first step is for participants to consciously connect their breathing with vocal emission. As obvious as it may seem, many people forget to breathe before speaking. These initial exercises will help the group familiarize themselves with this vital mechanism while also allowing them to appreciate the regulatory effects of healthy breathing and phonation on their autonomic state. Making vowel sounds is a widely practiced warm-up before singing. The chosen sequence optimizes the harmonics of each vowel, producing an intense vibration. Here are your instructions for the group:

- Sit or stand in a comfortable position. Your back should be straight but not stiff, with shoulders well below your ears. Soften your jaw, let your tongue fall, and relax your lips. Imagine separating your eyes, flattening the space that connects them to the center of your forehead. Soften your gaze.
- Inhale deeply (as practiced in the previous session) and, on the exhale, open your mouth wide and say the sound "uh" (as in ugly). Hold it for the duration of your exhale. Repeat this action three or four times.
- Do the same thing, now, using the "eh", as in bed.
- Experiment, now, with the sounds "ee" (as in tree), "aw" (as in awe), "oo" (as in blue). The "ee" sound (as in tree) should make you naturally smile. Consciously inhale before producing each sound, and stop when you run out of breath.
- Finally, explore the entire vowel sequence. Notice how you change the position of your mouth to make each sound.

This exercise usually lasts about eight minutes. At the conclusion, encourage the group to reflect on the activity's impact.

Exercise 2 – Making Sounds: U-O and VU*

After familiarizing ourselves with the basic mechanism "inhalation, phonation", we move on to experimenting with the sounds U-O (sounds like "oo-oh") and Vuuu ("voo", rhymes with blue). Due to their ability to produce vibration, these sounds greatly benefit the vagus nerve (adapted from Peter Levine, 2005 – exercise shared during Somatic Experiencing training). Encourage the group to let the sounds flow as they come. It doesn't matter if they are out of tune, unsteady, or uncertain. There is no goal to achieve, no performance to give, no audience to impress. U-O and Vuuu can be anything: a mere sound, a cry for help, an expression of pain, satisfaction, or happiness: whatever feels right and authentic. Lead them through the following activity:

- Sit or stand in a comfortable position. Your back should be straight but not stiff, with shoulders dropped well below your ears. Soften your jaw, let your tongue fall, and relax your lips. Imagine separating your eyes, flattening the space that connects them to the center of your forehead. Soften your gaze.
- Inhale and, as you breathe out, softly pronounce the sound VUUUUUUU... Keep it going, holding it until you run out of breath. Try to notice the vibration in your mouth, throat, chest, and stomach. You might even feel it in your limbs. It is a healing vibration that fosters self-regulation. Repeat the cycle four or five times.
- Now, do the same for the sound UUU-OOOOOO. Let it flow as you exhale until you run out of breath. If you wish, place your hand on your throat to feel the vibration of the sound under your fingers.
- Repeat the cycle four or five times.

Give the group five to six minutes to do this exercise. When they have finished, remind them to check how they feel afterward.

Exercise 3 – Chanting: The Traditional Mantras Aum and Sat Nam*

Chanting involves the rhythmic utterance of words or simple phrases over a narrow range of notes. This repetition has a sort of hypnotic and lulling effect on the nervous system.

Many spiritual traditions feature chanting mantras. But what are mantras? They first appeared in the *Vedas*, the oldest scriptures in Hinduism. The word derives from Sanskrit and consists of two syllables: *man*, which stands for *the one who thinks*, that is, man, and *tra*, which means *to protect, save, preserve*. Therefore, mantras serve the purpose of providing succor, refuge, and direction to the mind. Recited for millennia, they are considered powerful, healing, and sacred, acting as a passkey, an access code to specific states of consciousness.

We will begin our experimentation by chanting two traditional mantras: Aum (pronounced "omm") and Sat Nam (Figure 7.3). The Aum was originally a Hindu symbol of the Absolute, equivalent to *the one who creates, guards and destroys the universe*. It has been incorporated into various meditative and yogic traditions to represent primordial sound. Sat Nam is practiced in Kundalini yoga and means: *I salute and worship the divine, the only truth; it is in everything and everything is in it*. Reciting these mantras strengthens the cardiovascular system, fortifies the diaphragm, and conditions the voice box. Introduce the activity as follows:

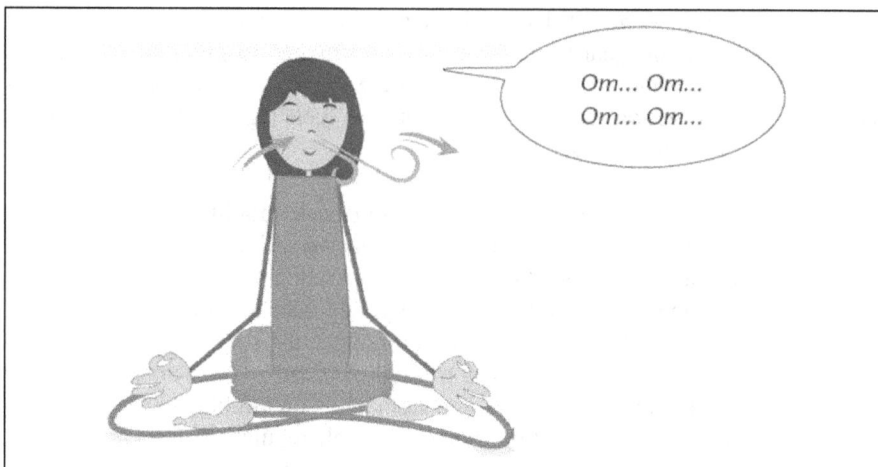

Figure 7.3 Chanting Traditional Mantras: Om and Sat Nam.

- Stay in the same position you used for the previous exercise; keep your back straight, shoulders open and relaxed. Close your eyes or look down, softening your jaw and lips.
- Inhale deeply and, as you exhale, pronounce the syllable Om. Open your mouth wide during the O, like a yawn, and bring your lips together for the M without clenching your teeth. Feel the sound vibrating between your upper and lower incisors. Hold the sound for as long as your breath allows, gradually letting it fade away.
- Experiment with various pitches until you find *your* OM, the sound that will make you feel comfortable and vibrate effortlessly as if it were singing itself. This process activates the membranes of your lungs, promoting better air exchange and increasing the oxygen level in the blood. Continue like this, breathing in and chanting the OM mantra 11 times.
- Now, let's move on to Sat Nam. This mantra differs from Om because it involves thinking the syllable Sat on the inhale and producing the sound Nam on the exhale. Follow the above instructions and repeat the cycle 11 times in a row.

The exercise lasts about 8 minutes in total. As always, encourage participants to look inward to fully grasp the impact of the activity.

Exercise 4 – Chanting: Mantras for the Third Millennium

Alongside traditional mantras, we can recite formulas that are applicable to the moment we are living in, our needs, and our sensibilities. Beyond the yoga mat or meditation cushion, our mantras can be chanted in everyday life, whenever we carry a burden on our hearts, feel fragile and need comfort, or when we are anxious or upset. We can chant them silently in our minds, recite them, sing them out loud, or write them down. The speed at which we say them will depend on their length. Short mantras – one to three syllables – should be repeated more slowly than longer ones. The pitch of the sound can vary from person to person and from time to time. The goal is to discover our unique way of chanting the mantras. Practicing them freely enables us to savor their energizing or calming effects without our mind wandering or becoming numb.

Here are some examples of mantras for the third millennium:

- *I'm safe here.*
- *It is part of a larger design.*
- *I can count on me.*
- *My heart knows.*
- *I won't let emotions take over; I can breathe them out.*
- *I can let go of what hurt me.*
- *I'm not my thoughts, and my thoughts aren't me.*
- *This moment is forever, this moment is all I have.*
- *I breathe in serenity, I breathe out serenity.*
- *I love joy, and joy loves me.*

• Read the list a few times and identify the mantra that speaks to you at this moment.
• Take up the position you used for the previous exercises and take a few seconds to center yourself.
• Recite the mantra you have chosen 11 times, observing what happens to your mind and body during the repetition.

At the end of the exercise, prompt participants to turn their attention inward and reflect on how reciting the mantra impacted them.

Exercise 5 – Chanting: Quiet Mind Mantras*

Along the lines of the previous exercise, here are two mantras that we developed, reinterpreting the traditional repertoire (see Figure 7.4). You can choose whether to propose one, the other, or both. The first step is to provide a model. Chant or sing the mantra for the group so they can learn it by heart. After making sure that the group can recite it correctly, lead the chant, providing the following instructions:

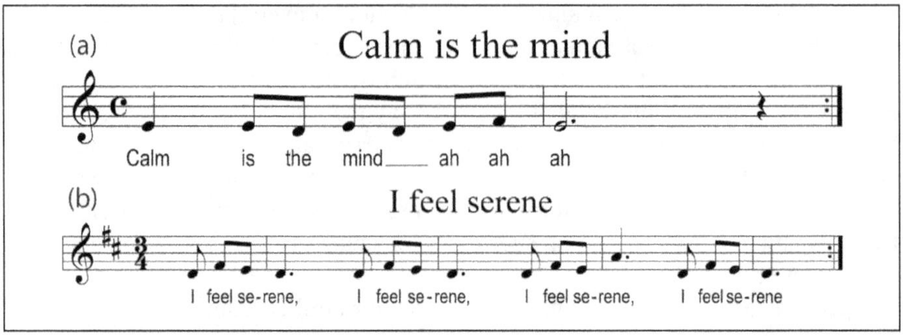

Figure 7.4 (a) and (b) Singing Mantras.

• Get into position (the one you used in the previous exercises) and take a moment to center yourself.
• Chant the mantra, always taking care to inhale before producing the sound.
• Repeat the sequence 11 times.

As always, conclude by encouraging participants to focus inward on the impact of chanting.

Exercise 6 – Chanting: To Each Their Own

A mantra serves as an affirmation. It should always possess a unique energy, a particular value for those who recite it. You can get creative and come up with your own formulas, touching on a wide variety of topics. The only constraint is to keep it short. Mantras should not consist of more than seven or eight words at most. Ask participants to devise their own. It may be a phrase that has meaning for them or words that make them feel calm, connected, or uplifted.

• Spend some time crafting your mantra, ensuring it produces a specific effect on your mind, body, and spirit. Choose each sound, letter, and word carefully.
• Once you have created your formula, get into position and give yourself a moment to center yourself.
• Recite the mantra you have created 11 times, noticing its effect throughout.

Afterward, prompt the group to reflect on how chanting their mantra impacted their body and mind.

Exercise 7 – Humming: Happy Birthday

Humming is the act of making a sound or melody with your mouth closed. Bee Breathing, which we experienced in the previous session, is an example of humming. It involves keeping your lips relaxed and picturing the sound moving forward. The sensation should be that of holding an air-filled balloon between the teeth.

Why is humming beneficial for the vagus nerve? Because it generates a vibration that spreads from the throat throughout the entire skull. It is a healing sound: it alleviates stress, lowers blood pressure, and improves lymphatic circulation. Suggest a familiar melody for the group to hum – like "Happy Birthday". Any song will do, as long as everyone knows it. Lead the group through this exercise with the following instructions:

- Get into position and take a moment to center yourself.
- Inhale and, on the exhale, hum *Happy Birthday to you...* and so on.
- Stop when you're out of breath, inhale, and start back from where you left off.

At the end of the activity, as always, encourage participants to focus their attention on the internal impact of humming.

Exercise 8 – Singing: Hey Jude

Singing produces remarkable physical and emotional benefits. Singing our favorite song – "With or Without You", "Imagine", "Hey Jude", whatever – at the top of your lungs is an exhilarating experience. But for all intents and purposes, it also functions as a form of exercise. When we sing, whether we are aware of it or not, we breathe deeply, coordinate our breathing with our vocal output, and engage as many muscles as we use during a run. Our voice box gets a workout, our lungs and diaphragm are activated, and the heart pumps blood. But there's more. With or without musical accompaniment, our bodies act as instruments. Sound flows through us, produced by that vibration that radiates from the throat into the body, massaging the vagus nerve, whose warm and reassuring energy soothes us.

Music is an art form capable of putting us in touch with our most authentic and profound emotional core. When we sing together – be it in a band or choir – we create a socially unifying experience, working towards a common goal. Notes become our shared vocabulary. Neuroception interprets this process as a safety cue. Our physiology responds by producing an intense sense of connection to ourselves and others. We feel secure, joyful, interdependent, and co-regulated by each other (Figure 7.5).

If you are not a musician, don't play an instrument, and are worried about leading the group in a singing activity, rest assured there are countless ways to approach this. The simplest is to sing without accompaniment. If you want to take it a step further, today, the internet provides us with thousands of free karaoke music tracks. Find one before class, ensure all the participants know the song, and use that.

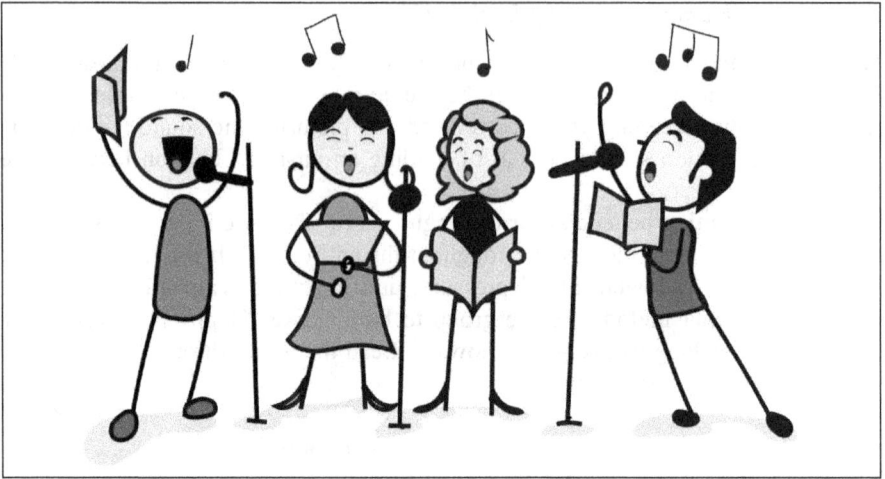

Figure 7.5 Singing or Playing Together Can Be a Powerful and Regulating Experience for the Nervous System.

Project the song lyrics or distribute them as a handout, then give the group the following instructions:

- Get into position again, relaxed but keeping your back straight. Make sure your jaw is unclenched and your lips loose.
- Soon you will hear the opening notes of the song we selected (*if you are using a backing track or accompanying yourself with an instrument*). We are all going to sing together. This is not a performance. There is no audience to impress. We don't have to be *good*. We sing as we know how to do it. We sing for the joy of doing it. We sing for fun, life, and togetherness, giving voice to the flame that shines inside us.

If you are using a backing track, start it and lead the group in song. As always, at the end of the exercise, remind participants to turn their attention inward and savor the resonance left by the activity.

Exercise 9 – Prosody

As mentioned above, prosody refers to the stress, tempo, and intonation of vocal output. In neuroceptive terms, the overall musicality of the spoken voice is a powerful indicator of safety or danger. This exercise gives the group the opportunity to explore the impact of prosody on their autonomic landscape. Participants will be experimenting with intonation, rhythm, and volume. Prepare a list of short,

everyday sentences beforehand (e.g., *Come here. What are you doing? Wait...*).
Then, read these, giving the following instructions:

- Center yourself and turn your attention inward.
- Notice everything that happens to you – in your body, your mind, your emotions – when you hear: "Come here!" (*imperative tone*). Observe how your body and mind respond.

After a pause of about 20 seconds, repeat the same phrase, giving your voice a different intonation to convey pleading, comfort, or criticism. In other words, change your prosody. Ask the group to notice how they respond to the different intonations. Repeat the pattern with all selected phrases. At the end of the exercise, gather the group and start a discussion about what they observed.

Exercise 10 – Words That Frighten, Words That Calm

Our neuroceptive surveillance system is so finely tuned that even listening to or reading individual words can elicit feelings of safety or danger and mobilize an autonomic reaction. Consider how evocative terms like "love", "joy", "happiness", "freedom", "travel", and "friendship" convey warmth, while others like "death", "haste", "blood", "work", "hatred", "war", and "massacre" induce tension. In the following exercise, you will guide the group in exploring linguistic triggers capable of mobilizing protective responses, followed by a list of terms that could anchor them to the reassuring energy of the ventral vagal system. Give participants the following instructions:

- Take a moment. Turn your attention inward.
- Give your mind's eye permission to flip through the pages of an imaginary dictionary or scroll through a list of words.
- Let your attention rest on those words that put you on edge, bringing you into a state of mobilization/immobilization.
- Write down your list.
- Now reread the words one at a time, paying attention to the autonomic state they send you to.
- Let these *words that frighten you* slip away, fade out. Focus on the *words that calm you*, those capable of generating ventral vagal energy within you. Write down your list.
- Reread the words one at a time, paying attention to the way the experience of security and connection is expressed in your body when listening to these terms.

At the end of the exercise, start a short exchange with the participants, pooling their impressions and comments.

Exercise 11 – I Listen, Therefore I Feel...

We have come to the last experiential part of today's meeting, the one dedicated to listening. First of all, how do we *hear*? We perceive the vibrations in the air that, captured by the eardrum, travel to our inner ear. This stimulates the vagus nerve, which is why even just listening to certain sounds can enhance our vagal tone. For example, the sounds of Aum or Sat Nam mantras (which we explored in Exercise 3) are known to calm the heart, regularize breathing, and lower blood pressure in most people.

Listening means getting in touch with the outside world by tuning in to the rich, varied, and diversified sound environment surrounding us. Our nervous system constantly receives sounds – both artificial and natural – that it interprets as cues capable of inducing specific autonomic states. Some sounds fade into the background, ignored by our neuroception due to their familiarity or neutrality, while others evoke fear or tranquility. And, finally, we come to music. In a much more complex and nuanced way than a single sound, music can *make us feel* a certain way. Typically, rock energizes, classical relaxes, folk uplifts, and meditative music soothes, while the soundtrack of a horror movie keeps us on the edge of our seats. But be careful not to generalize. We have seen how neuroception is shaped by experience, and this also applies to our musical tastes. Someone might get irritated listening to Tibetan bells, while someone else might find rock boring. There is, however, a common denominator which concerns us all and transcends our individual preferences: when we listen to music, our nervous system tends to remain in an optimal activation state. We can be fully alive without being mobilized, and fully emotional or vulnerable without immobilizing or shutting down.

We can explore the world of sound and its effects on our nervous system through a series of activities. The first exposes participants to various stimuli and asks them to study the type of autonomic response produced by each. Download the audio track we made for this purpose from the online resources or create your own sound compilation. If you want to create your own playlist, just keep in mind that each track should last no more than 20 or 30 seconds. This is enough time to stimulate our autonomic nervous system and investigate its reactions. Below is a list of possible sound inputs:

- Traffic noise.
- The chirping of birds.
- The cry of a baby.
- The drumming of rain (Figure 7.6).
- Ocean waves.
- An excerpt of classical music.
- An excerpt of rock music.

Lead the listening experience by providing the following instructions:

- Take a moment to turn your attention inward.
- I am about to play you a series of sounds, each different from the last. Whenever the audio track stops, observe how your nervous system responds. Take a mental note of your reactions.

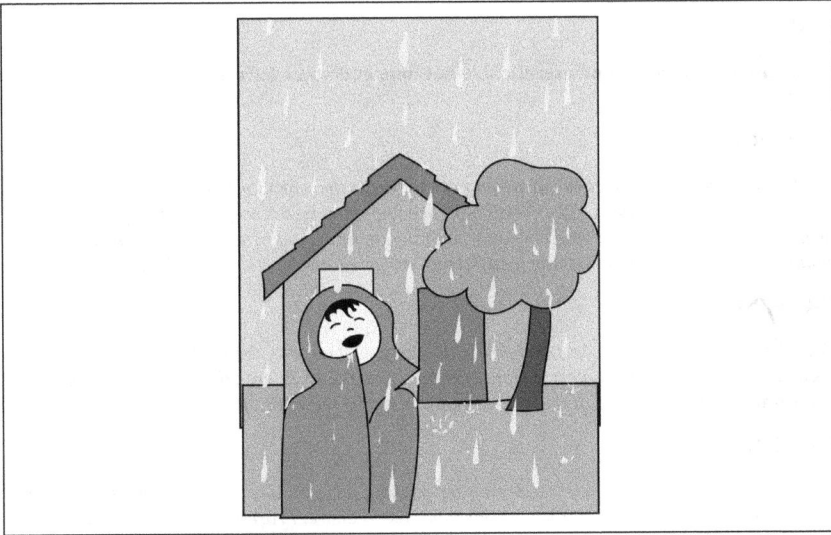

Figure 7.6 I Listen, Therefore I Feel.

At the end of the activity, bring the group back together and collect their feedback.

7.4   Setting Homework

The Sound that Suits You

It's time to present the homework of the week (Figure 7.7 illustrates an example of a homework assignment from a course participant.). Provide each group member with a handout describing all the exercises covered in session, so they can practice at home. Share the following instructions:

> Throughout today's session, you have experimented with various activities related to sound. Using the handouts, go over and repeat the exercises we did in class as often as possible at home. Identify the three activities that are most meaningful to you. Answer the following questions in writing:
>
> • What are your favorite activities?
> • How did these exercises impact your nervous system?
> • How did you feel after doing them?
>
> Also, listen intentionally. Take notice of sounds from nature, classical music, sacred music, electronic music, jazz, punk, rock, film soundtracks, jingles, etc. Develop the habit of recognizing which parts of your nervous system respond to the sounds you hear.

MARTIN

What are my favorite sound exercises? What impact do they have on my autonomic nervous system?

MANTRAS

The OM mantras helps me concentrate and relax, due to the vibrations in my chest and throat, as well as the slow and prolonged exhalation, accompanied by the sensation of emptying my lungs. This is useful for relieving tension when I am in the sympathetic state. With the SAT NAM mantra, I had a harder time staying focused for longer, as my mind wandered easily.

U-O and VU

The vibrations in my upper chest and throat, the long exhales, and the U-O and VU vocalizations allow me to achieve a state of rest, although less intense than with the Om mantra. The vibrating pronunciation of the vowel sounds also has the same effect on me.

BEE BREATHING

An example of humming I use is bee breathing. Making this sound relaxes me. Chanting doesn't have a positive effect on me because it feels more like a chore. I rarely use singing, only when I am already in a ventral vagal state, so I can stay there longer.

LISTENING TO SOUNDS

The sound of the ocean has the power to calm my autonomic nervous system. A stormy sea activates me but not in the sympathetic state: it is not a feeling of danger, it is more an activation of the senses and a greater feeling of being present. The rustle of the wind in the leaves of big trees gives me a feeling of well-being and brings me into a ventral vagal state. The sounds of a thunderstorm have an invigorating effect on me, especially when combined with the smell of wet earth and air.

SOPHIA

What are my favorite sound exercises? What impact do they have on my autonomic nervous system?

LISTENING TO SOUNDS

The sounds that usually relax and calm me are the sounds produced by nature, such as the song of cicadas in summer, the sound of the waves, especially when I am on a boat, and the whistle of the wind. Music also has this calming and relaxing power, especially jazz, such as Frank Sinatra, and singers like Bruce Springsteen, because they take me back to my childhood.

MANTRAS

Mantras, on the other hand, recharge me in a particular way. The ones I use the most are: 'I'm full of resources and potential', 'I'm the architect of my own destiny', 'I love myself', and 'Post nubila Phoebus'. The latter is a phrase that my Latin teacher used to say a lot in high school, and it still has a strong energizing power, especially when I experience a disappointment.

Figure 7.7 Sound: Examples of Homework Filled Out by Course Participants.

7.5   Closing Ritual and Farewell

End the meeting by expressing gratitude to all participants' nervous systems. As you bid them farewell, encourage them to use sound as a regulating resource as often as possible.

Session 8

Movement

We have reached the final experiential session of the program. In previous meetings, the group experienced the regulatory potential of breath, and explored sound as both a safety or danger signal and a tool for autonomic nervous system modulation. Today, we will focus on another powerful instrument that directly influences the vagus nerve: movement. Engaging in activities together – a constant feature of this journey – should have fostered an environment of cooperation and exchange. The group feels connected and united. The aim is for participants to forge bonds and actively appreciate the power of relationships through their experiences on the course itself.

Learning Goals

- Reinforcing the idea that sound can function both as an indicator of safety or danger and a tool for autonomic regulation through the sharing of homework.
- Understanding the importance of movement as a tool for directly affecting vagus nerve function.
- Exploring a set of exercises and establishing a well-being routine centered on mindful movement.

Session Framework

1. Session opening and homework review – 60 minutes
2. Polyvagal Module 8 – 20 minutes
3. Experiential learning – 60 minutes
4. Setting homework – 10 minutes
5. Closing ritual and farewell – 5 minutes

N.B.: The times indicated are only intended as a guide. The process should be adapted to the group's needs, which we encourage you to prioritize as part of your roadmap.

DOI: 10.4324/9781003560968-13

8.1   Session Opening and Homework Review

After a warm welcome, the instructor will give a short summary of the previous session and comment on the homework submissions. Invite the group to actively note each other's experiences. This will enrich the range of possible situations in which sound can be used for modulating the autonomic nervous system.

8.2   Polyvagal Module 8

Before leading the day's activities, introduce the session's theme. Polyvagal Module 8 focuses on the close relationship between the activation of the autonomic nervous system and the resulting bodily responses. Emphasize the massive regulatory benefits of incorporating the practice of conscious movement into daily life. Use this script as a guide:

In the various stages of this journey of discovery we have been on together, we have seen how quickly the body responds to our autonomic states. This happens extremely quickly, even before we can process our feelings or understand what is happening to us. Our heart, our blood pressure, our breathing, and our muscles react instantaneously to the signals of safety or danger we detect within us, in the external environment, or in our relationships with others. Observing, paying attention to our body, learning to perceive it from the inside and interpret its responses is therefore a fundamental step in the development of autonomic awareness. This way, we will be able to map our activation states and learn to discern, moment by moment, where we are on our Autonomic Ladder.

However, the body is not merely a source of discomfort, the predestined target of our attack/escape or shutdown/collapse responses. The body is, in fact, the home of the Self. In other words, our body is us. By nurturing it, forging a relationship with it, listening, and tending to our physical state, we can transform our body into the cradle of our well-being, the temple of the most vital expression of ourselves.

One effective strategy for fostering a new way of inhabiting our skin is through practicing mindful movement (Figure 8.1). During today's session, we will engage in a series of physical exercises that allow us to tone our vagus nerve, as if it were a muscle. We will discover how this type of activity can help modulate our autonomic state and train our nervous system to bask in warm and relaxed ventral vagal energy. The goal for you is to develop a routine, making these exercises part of your daily self-care. Performing them regularly empowers you to take charge of your own healing and take back the reins of your life.

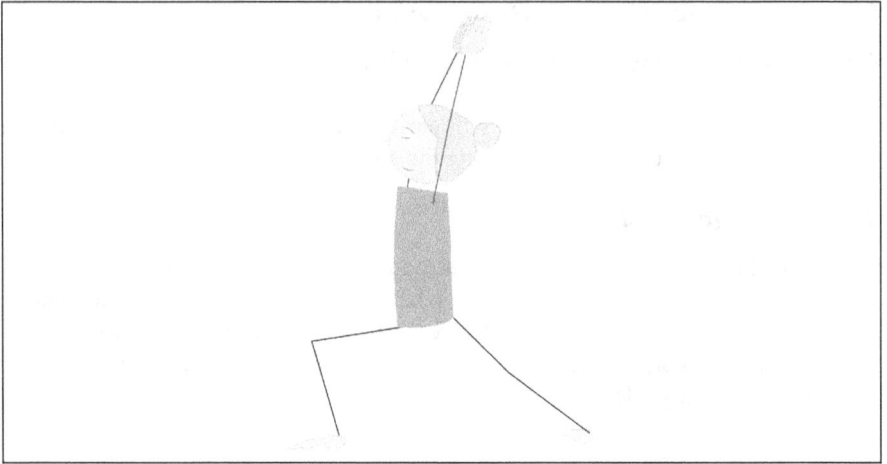

Figure 8.1 The Body Is the Home of Our Self.

8.3   Experiential Activities

The experiential section of this module involves movement exercises drawn mainly from Hatha yoga, a type of practice recognized for its highly therapeutic potential for the nervous system.

Before starting, the instructor must set up the workspace. If the program is conducted in person, mats should be laid on the floor, and cushions or meditation benches should be provided if desired. If you are teaching online, ensure your participants have their own ready and can adjust the video camera and settings so that everyone can see each other while performing the exercises.

Remind the group that a critical aspect of self-care is awareness of one's limits and the importance of not pushing too hard. If you like, you can reinforce this concept by recounting the story of *Goldilocks and The Three Bears*:

Goldilocks was, as her name suggests, a little girl with golden curls. One morning, she went for a walk in the forest. She caught a glimpse of a pretty wooden house among the trees and, driven by curiosity, decided to let herself in. Once there, Goldilocks found herself in a huge kitchen. In the middle of it stood a large table laden with several bowls of different sizes full of porridge. She sat down at the head of the table, with the largest bowl in front of her. Taking it in her hands, she thought, "This bowl is too big for me! There's far too much porridge here". She put the bowl back down and then moved to the other side of the table, where there was a tiny, tiny bowl. Goldilocks picked it up and thought, "This bowl is too small for me! There is not enough porridge here". Undaunted, she began to move from one table setting to another until she found the bowl just right for her: neither too big nor too small; not too much porridge nor too little, but just enough to satisfy her hunger.

Emphasize that the essence of conscious movement practice consists, first and foremost, of tuning into one's own bodily experience. Sometimes, this might also mean knowing when to stop and to push no further.

As always, when conducting activities, demonstrate the positions. If you are teaching in person, participate alongside the group. If online, ensure that all participants are performing the asanas correctly.

Highlight the connection between movement and breathing. Give the group the experience of these intertwined regulatory resources and help them savor their benefits. Extend a loving invitation to make the practice a personal journey, reminding them they can always make choices based on their nervous system's needs. Provide guidance in a non-directive manner, using invitations like:

- You can keep your eyes open or closed.
- Choose what feels best for you at this moment.
- Notice what type of breathing best anchors your nervous system to the energy of safety and connection in this pose.
- Feel free to personalize this asana in a way that works for you.

The proposed sequence offers targeted interventions that aim to follow the trajectory of the vagus nerve along the body: from the head, through the neck, along the chest, and into the abdomen. Each pose will gently stimulate and tone the nerve's various branches, rejuvenating the nervous system as a whole. It starts with the Mountain Pose asana, which typically serves as the gateway to the practice.

Lead the activities without rushing, allowing participants to savor the effects moment by moment. After all, yoga is mindfulness in action. Remind the group not only to *do* but also to *feel* and *observe* while doing. The asanas have a profound effect on both our inner universe and our physical dimension. Pausing and paying attention is key: this is where conscious movement becomes transformative, leading to peace, serenity, and joy.

As always, choose the exercises that suit you from those below. Tailor your sequence to your sensibilities and, above all, to the unique needs of the group you are leading.

Exercise 1 – Mountain Pose (Tadasana)

This asana is simple to perform but represents an extraordinary opportunity to intimately connect with our breathing and physical sensations. Mountain Pose also allows us to ground ourselves. Planting our feet firmly makes us more stable (Figure 8.2) and ready for anything.

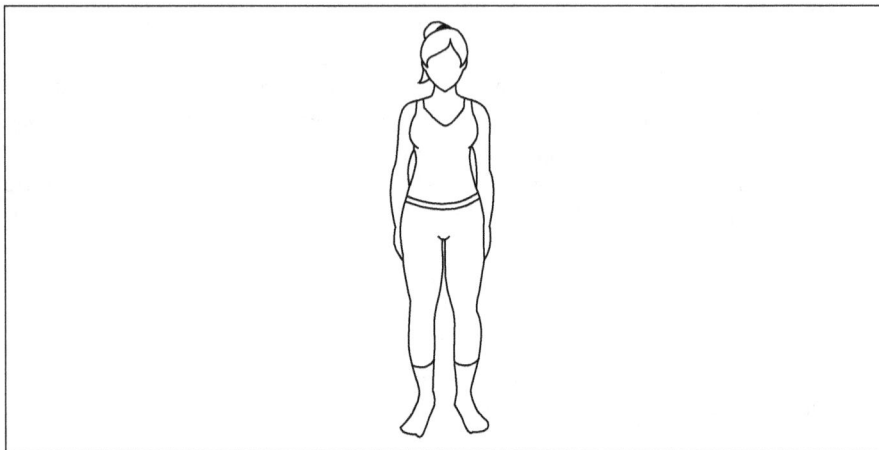

Figure 8.2 Mountain Pose.

- Starting from an upright position, spread your feet a hip-width apart, parallel with each other.
- Begin to feel the weight of your body pushing downwards, through your legs, until it reaches the heels and soles of your feet.
- Allow your back to rise upwards. Lift from your waist, following your body's natural curvature. Keep your chest open, shoulders relaxed and slightly back, and your arms loose at your sides, fingers pointing down, and palms facing your thighs.
- Now, find your center. With your eyes closed, rock gently back and forth until you feel deeply rooted to the ground. Remain in this position for four or five breathing cycles, observing how your body responds to this asana.

Exercise 2 – Salamander Pose

This exercise can be performed either standing or sitting (Figure 8.3), depending on each participant's preference.

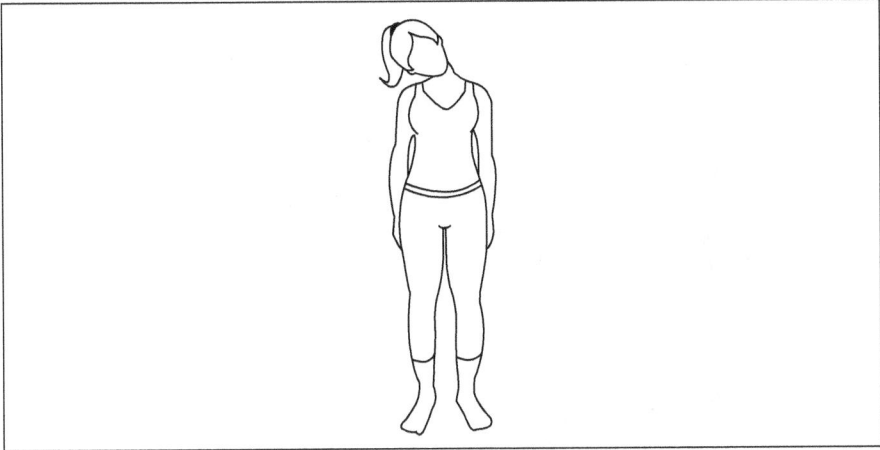

Figure 8.3 Salamander Pose.

- Start in Mountain Pose. If standing is challenging, you can sit at the edge of your chair with your feet firmly planted on the floor. Remember to relax your shoulders and open your chest. Your arms should be loose, and your hands should rest on your thighs. Your neck should follow its natural curvature, and your gaze should point straight in front of you.
- Inhale, and on the exhale gently bend your neck, bringing your left ear closer to your left shoulder. Keep your shoulders down and your gaze forward.
- Inhale, and on the exhale bring your head back to the center.
- Inhale, and on the exhale gently bend your neck, bringing your right ear closer to your right shoulder. Keep your shoulders down and your gaze forward.
- Inhale, and on the exhale bring your head back to the center.

Get them to repeat the entire sequence – tilting the head to the left and then the right – five times. A variation of this exercise (Rosenberg, 2017) involves holding each position for 60 seconds.

Exercise 3 – Turning the Head

This exercise is similar to the Salamander Pose, but here the focus is on turning the head rather than tilting it. It can also be performed standing or sitting (Figure 8.4).

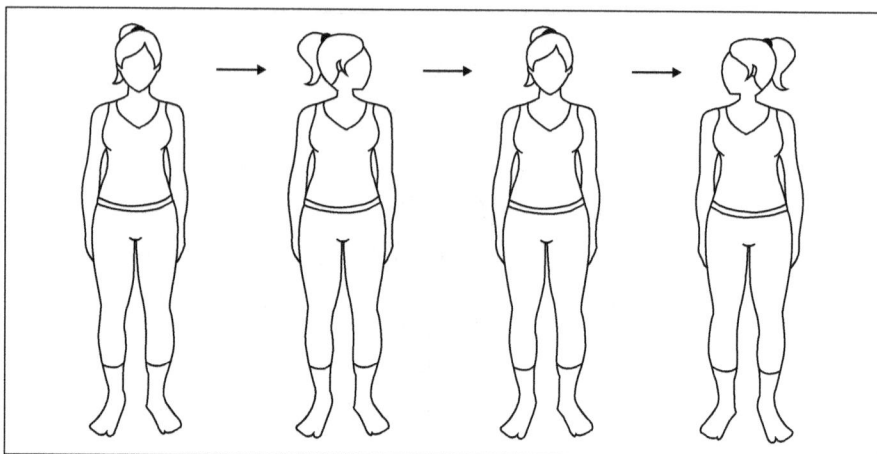

Figure 8.4 Turning the Head.

- Begin with Mountain Pose. Whether standing or sitting, keep your shoulders relaxed and away from your ears, your chest open, your arms relaxed, and your hands resting softly on your thighs. Your neck should follow its natural curvature, and your gaze should be straight ahead.
- Inhale, and on the exhale turn your chin towards your left shoulder, without lifting it. Your gaze should follow.
- Inhale, and on the exhale return your chin back to the center and your gaze towards the front.
- Inhale, and on the exhale turn your chin towards your right shoulder. Do not lift it. Your gaze should follow.
- Inhale, and on the exhale return your chin back to the center and your gaze towards the front.
- Repeat the entire sequence, turning the head to the left and right, five times.

Exercise 4 – The Gaze

Exercising the eyes is considered highly beneficial for the vagus nerve. These movements allow the muscles at the base of the skull to relax, reducing the tension in the nerve. It also improves blood circulation.

Invite the participants to sit down. The ideal position for this exercise involves interlacing the hands behind the head, resting them at the base of the neck, while keeping the elbows wide apart. If this posture feels uncomfortable, participants could simply keep their heads upright. After all group members have identified their starting position, provide the following instructions (Figure 8.5):

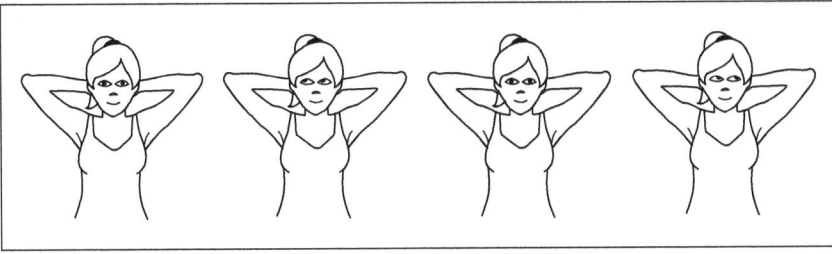

Figure 8.5 The Gaze.

- Keep your head still, your shoulders well open and relaxed.
- Direct your eyes up towards your left eyebrow and, breathing consciously, hold this position for five breathing cycles.
- Still without moving your head, now turn your eyes towards your right eyebrow. Hold this position for five breathing cycles.
- Bring your gaze back towards the front, noting the impact of exercise on your mind and body.

Exercise 5 – Shoulder Rolls (Skanda Chakra Asana)

This exercise can be performed either standing or sitting (Figure 8.6).

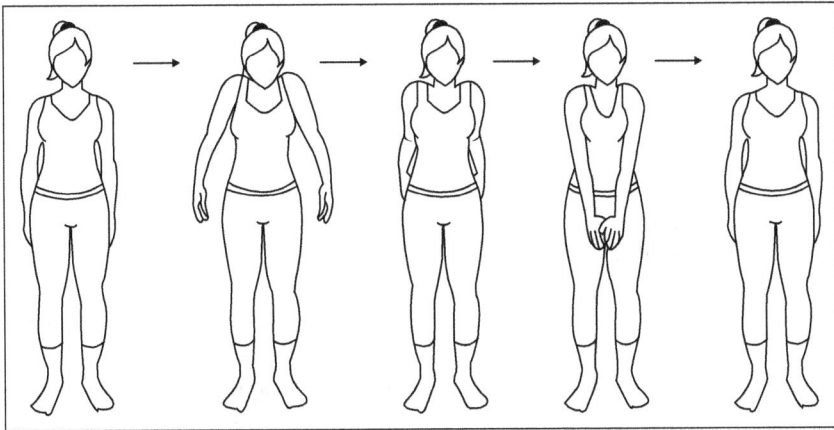

Figure 8.6 Shoulder Rolls.

- Begin in Mountain Pose. Whether standing or sitting, make sure your shoulders are relaxed and away from your ears, your chest is open, and your arms are loose. Your neck follows its natural curvature, and your gaze is straight ahead.
- Inhaling, bring your shoulders up to your ears and then roll them behind you.

- On the exhale, first push your shoulders gently downwards and then move them forward, until they make a complete rotation. It might help to think of drawing large circles in the air, as if your shoulders were a paintbrush.
- After completing five rolls in one direction, reverse it. Roll your shoulders from front to back, allowing the movement to become progressively smoother.

Exercise 6 – Standing Crescent Pose (Indudalasana)

This exercise can be done standing (Figure 8.7) or sitting.

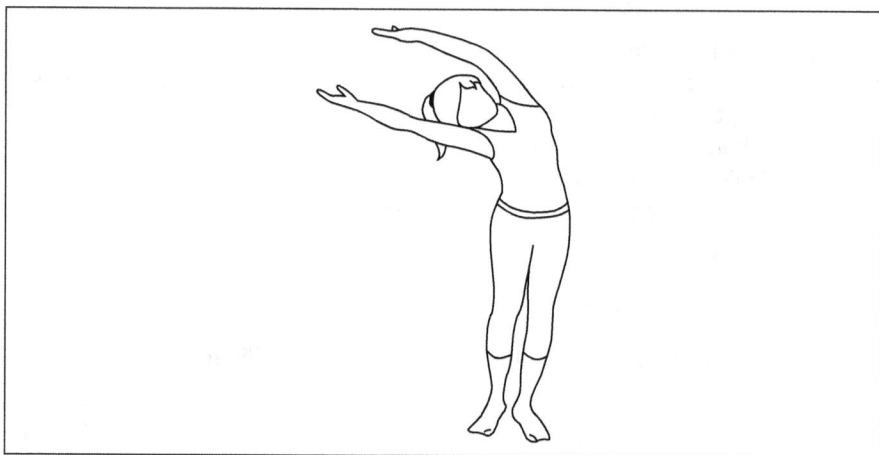

Figure 8.7 Standing Crescent Pose.

- Start in Mountain Pose. Whether standing or sitting, ensure your shoulders are relaxed and away from your ears, your chest is open, and your arms are loose. Your neck should follow its natural curvature, and your gaze should be straight ahead.
- As you inhale, raise your arms above your head as if you were trying to reach the moon above you.
- As you exhale, tilt your arms to the left, imagining that you are moving the moon you are holding in your hands to the other side. Breathe in the asana while extending the arms as far as you can to the left. Observe the quality of your breathing in this position and where you perceive it the most. Hold this pose for five full breathing cycles.
- Repeat the exercise to the right.

Exercise 7 – Standing Forward Bend (Uttanasana)

This exercise can also be performed standing (Figure 8.8) or sitting.

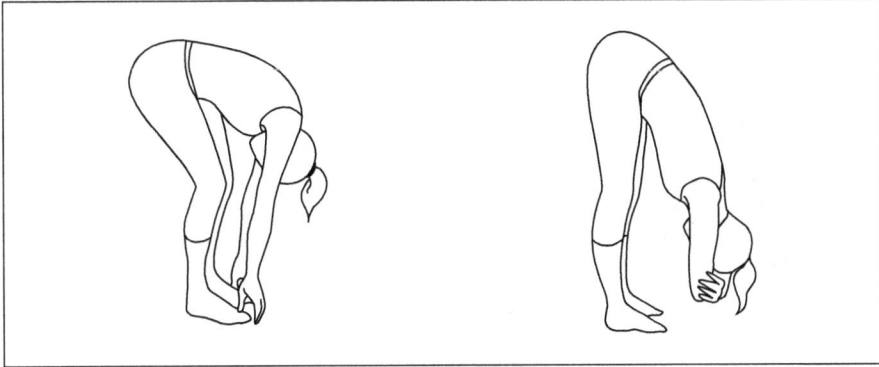

Figure 8.8 Standing Forward Bend.

- Begin in Mountain Pose. Whether standing or sitting, ensure your shoulders are relaxed and away from your ears, your chest is open, and your arms are loose. Your neck should follow its natural curvature, and your gaze should be straight ahead.
- Inhale, and on the exhale lean your arms and your entire body forward. Imagine you are a ragdoll or seaweed at the bottom of the sea. Your neck is relaxed but your head is heavy, pulling your torso towards the ground.
- If you want, cross your arms and cup your elbows in your hands, holding them as you press downward slightly. Gently swing them left and right, paying attention to the needs of your spine and nervous system.
- Stay in this position, getting gradually lower, for five complete breathing cycles. Notice everything you experience while holding this asana.
- If you have crossed your arms, release them now. Inhale and slowly rise back to an upright position. Keep your knees slightly bent and unroll your spine, one vertebra at a time. Your head is the last to arrive. Notice your spine as you regain your standing position. Take a moment to observe how your autonomic nervous system responds to this change in perspective.

Exercise 8 –Triangle Pose (Trikonasana)

This asana starts from a standing position (Figure 8.9).

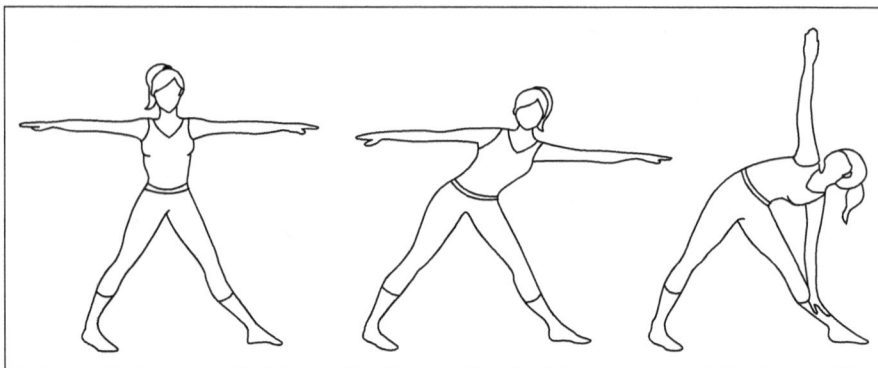

Figure 8.9 Triangle Pose.

- Begin in Mountain Pose.
- Inhale, and on the exhale take a wider stance, spreading your legs apart with your feet facing forward. At the same time, raise your arms to the sides until they reach shoulder height.
- Inhale, and on the exhale turn your left foot 45 degrees towards the side.
- Inhale, and on the exhale move your right hip to the right, twisting your torso and reaching down with your left hand to grab your left leg, calf, or ankle, wherever feels most comfortable. Keep your shoulders to the front, above your hips. Your right arm should be stretching upwards, with the palm of your hand facing the front.
- Inhale, and on the exhale turn your gaze towards the fingertips of your right hand.
- Stay in position and breathe consciously. Try to go lower, keeping your weight even, on the soles of both feet. Stay in the asana for five complete breathing cycles, savoring its effect.

Repeat the exercise on the other side.

Exercise 9 – Warrior Pose #1 (Virabhadrasana I)

This asana starts from a standing position (Figure 8.10).

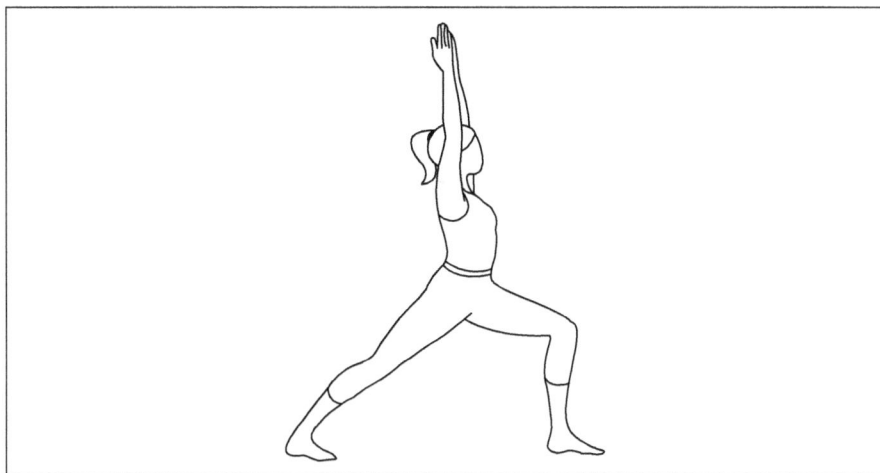

Figure 8.10 Warrior Pose #1.

- Enter Mountain Pose.
- Take a big step to the side to widen your stance. Keep your feet parallel in front of you.
- Rotate your right foot 90 degrees and your left foot 45 degrees, ensuring both heels stay aligned, standing on the same imaginary line. Turn your chest and abdomen to the right, so that you are looking towards your right leg.
- Raise your arms overhead, alongside your ears, with the palms of your hands facing inward, towards each other.
- Bend your right knee at a 90-degree angle in front of you, ensuring it aligns with your ankle without extending beyond your toes.
- Breathe into the position, going deeper, trying to place your weight evenly on both feet. The overall sensation should be one of pride and grounding. Tune into the bodily sensations, allowing them to guide you in balancing commitment and surrender. Hold this pose for five complete breaths, savoring its effects.
- Repeat on the opposite side.

Exercise 10 – Warrior Pose #2 (Virabhadrasana II)

This asana starts from a standing position (see Figure 8.11).

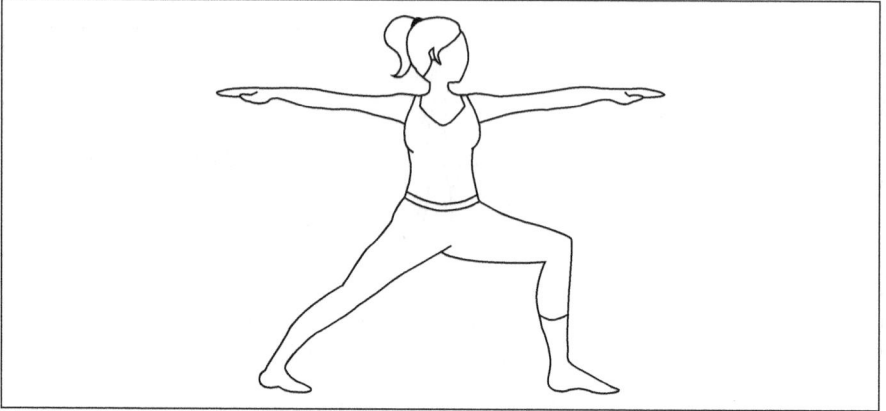

Figure 8.11 Warrior Pose #2.

- Begin in Mountain Pose.
- Take a step out to the side and spread your legs apart as far as possible, keeping your feet parallel.
- Rotate your right foot 90 degrees and your left foot 45 degrees, ensuring both heels stay aligned. Do not turn your chest and abdomen: keep in line with the long side of your mat.
- Square your shoulders with your hips. Now, raise your arms to shoulder height, with the palms of your hands facing down. Open your shoulders as best you can.
- Bend your right knee at a 90-degree angle in front of you. Your knee should remain in line with your ankle without extending beyond your toes. Do not rotate your torso – keep it square above your hips.
- Inhale, and on the exhale turn your gaze towards the middle finger of your right hand, keeping your arms horizontal. Hold the pose for five complete breathing cycles, going deeper every time. Listen to what is happening to your mind and body. If unpleasant feelings or critical comments emerge, observe them for what they are, maintaining a loving and accepting mindset.
- Repeat the exercise on the other side.

Exercise 11 – Cat–Cow (Bitilasana–Marjaryasana)

Begin the asana by getting on your hands and knees (Figure 8.12).

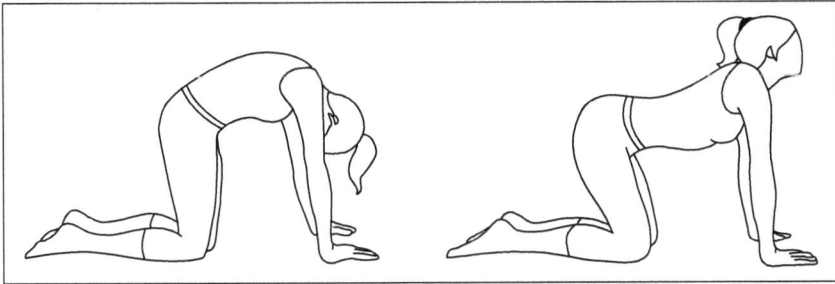

Figure 8.12 Cat–Cow.

- To make the Cat pose, kneel down, and bring your hands level with your shoulders. Plant them firmly on the ground. Your arms are extended, your knees open to the same width as your hips, and the tops of your feet are resting on the floor.
- As you breathe out, round your back upwards, as if you were a cat stretching, moving your tailbone towards the front of the mat while tucking your pelvis in and up. Allow your head to fall between your shoulders, gazing towards your legs.
- As you breathe in, transition into the Cow pose: arch your back downwards, lifting your tailbone and allowing your belly to drop towards the floor. Visualizing the shape of the cow's back may help. The highest points should be the top of your head and your tailbone.
- Repeat five times, letting your breath guide the timing and rhythm of your movements. Begin from your tailbone and allow the wave-like motion to travel through your body.
- Tune in to how your body responds, and note what happens to your autonomic nervous system as you move and breathe like this.

Exercise 12 – Downward Dog (Ado Mukha Svanasana)

Start the asana on your hands and knees (Figure 8.13).

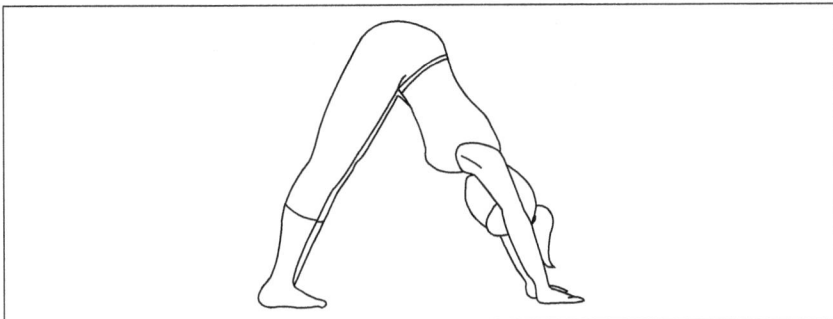

Figure 8.13 Downward Dog.

- For the Downward Dog pose, kneel down and place your hands on the ground at shoulder level. Your arms should be outstretched, your knees open to the same width as your hips, and your toes pressing on the ground.
- As you breathe in, extend your legs by planting your heels on the floor while lifting your knees off the mat and your pelvis upwards.
- As you breathe out, stretch your legs as far as you can, flattening your back while keeping your neck relaxed. Prioritize back stretch over leg extension.
- Keep breathing as you explore this pose. Try lifting one heel and then the other or taking small steps forward until you find a comfortable and stable position. Remain in the asana for five complete breathing cycles.

Exercise 13 – Cobra Pose (Bhujangasana)

This asana begins in a prone position, lying on your stomach, with your forehead touching the floor and arms at your sides (Figure 8.14).

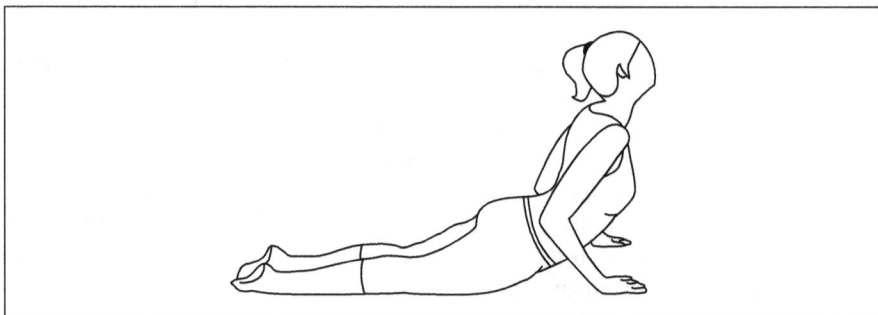

Figure 8.14 Cobra Pose.

- As you inhale and exhale, bring your legs together and press the tops of your feet to the floor.
- Keep breathing as you place your hands on the ground at shoulder height, allowing your shoulders to roll back and down as your chest spreads open while pressing down. Make sure your elbows are tucked in.
- Inhale and exhale, lifting your head, shoulders, and chest by engaging the muscles of your back and abdomen while pressing down on your hands. If comfortable, look upwards, but don't force the movement. Arch your back while keeping your abdominal muscles engaged. Go as far back as your spine allows, maintaining an open chest and relaxed shoulders and neck.
- Breathe into the position, go deeper. Stay in the asana for five complete breathing cycles, savoring its effect.

Exercise 14 – Sitting Spinal Twist (Parivrtta Sukhasana)

This twist begins in a seated position, either on a chair or cross-legged on the mat (Figure 8.15).

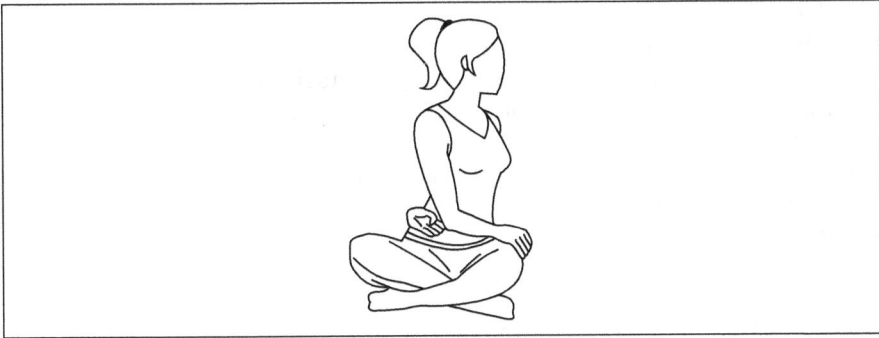

Figure 8.15 Sitting Spinal Twist.

- If using a chair, sit on the edge, away from the backrest. Your feet must be apart, parallel, and firmly planted on the ground. If you are on a mat, cross your legs. It may help to use a cushion or a meditation bench. Your back should be erect, your shoulders low and relaxed.
- Place your right hand on your left knee and your left hand behind you, resting it on the floor as you sit upright. If reaching back feels uncomfortable, leave your hand near your tailbone. Gaze forward while inhaling in this position.
- On the exhale, rotate your left shoulder backwards, letting your right shoulder follow. Allow your head to go along with this twist, bringing your chin and gaze towards your left shoulder.
- Hold this position for five full breathing cycles. Notice how your body and mind respond as you maintain the twist.
- Return to the center.
- Twist to the other side, holding the position for five full breathing cycles.

Exercise 15 – Supine Spinal Twist (Supta Matsyendrasana)

This asana (Figure 8.16) starts from the supine position, lying on your back.

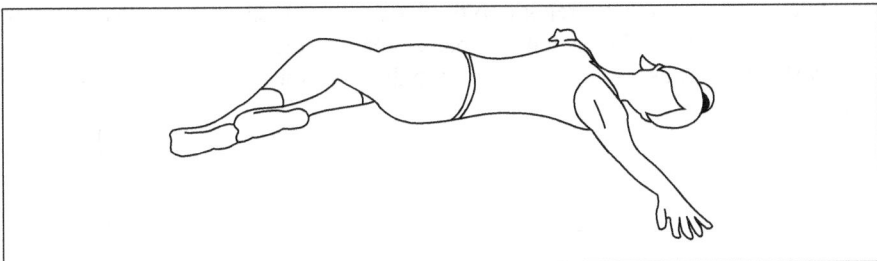

Figure 8.16 Supine Spinal Twist.

- Lie on your back with bent knees and your feet flat on the ground.
- Inhale, and on the exhale cross your left leg over your right. Move your hips to the left by about a hand's width.
- Inhale, and on the exhale bring your arms to shoulder height, making a cross shape.
- Inhale, and on the exhale let your knees fall to the right until you feel your weight mainly on your left side. Your spine should be twisted along its entire length without any effort. Your shoulder blades are on the floor and your chest is open. Stay in the pose for five complete breathing cycles, going deeper. Observe how twisting impacts your natural breathing. Tune into the sensations within your mind and body.
- Repeat on the other side.

Exercise 16 – Child Pose (Balasana)

This asana involves kneeling (Figure 8.17). If necessary, place a pillow between your buttocks and calves, and another between your abdomen and thighs.

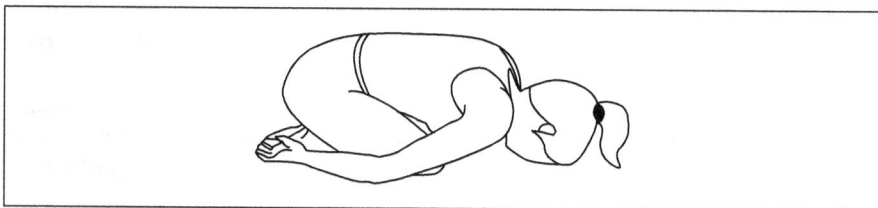

Figure 8.17 Child Pose.

- Start by sitting on your calves, with your buttocks resting on your heels. Your big toes should touch, and your knees should be slightly apart.
- Inhale, and as you exhale bend forward, letting your chest rest on your thighs. Your forehead should touch the floor with your arms placed alongside your body. Your weight should be on your heels, not your head. If you struggle to touch the ground with your forehead, consider using a yoga block or a pillow.
- Allow yourself to fully relax into the pose as you breathe, letting your breath flow naturally. Hold for ten complete breaths, observing how your internal world changes as you settle deeper into the position.

Exercise 17 – Lion Stretch

This exercise (Figure 8.18) starts from the supine position, lying on your back.

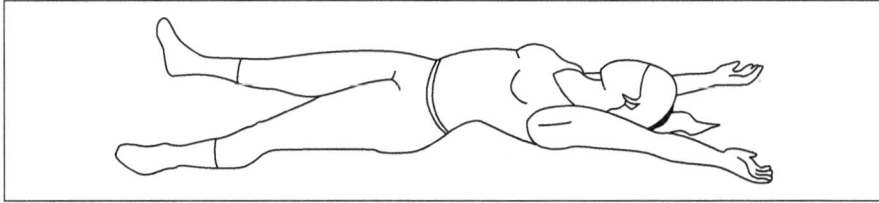

Figure 8.18 Lion Stretch.

- Lie on your back with your legs wide open and your big toes pointing outward. Keep your arms to your sides, slightly away from your trunk.
- Imagine that you are a lion waking up. Stretch as far as you can, bringing your arms above your head. You are yawning with your whole body, from the tips of your toes, up your legs, your trunk, your neck, your head, all the way to the tips of your fingers. After stretching, relax all your muscles.
- Repeat, alternating stretching and relaxing for three or four minutes.

Exercise 18 – Integration Pose (Shavasana)

This asana promotes full-body relaxation. It starts in the supine position. You can place a pillow under your knees, bending them slightly, to take the strain off your lower back if necessary (Figure 8.19).

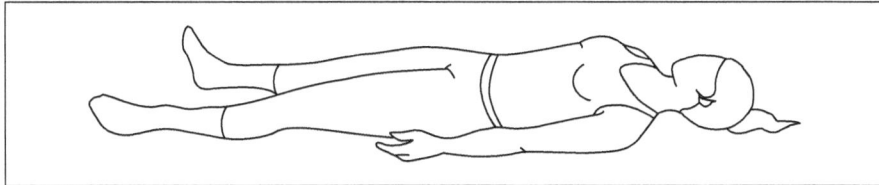

Figure 8.19 Integration Pose.

- Lie on your back with your legs wide open and your big toes pointing outward. Keep your arms to your sides, slightly away from your trunk.
- Allow your awareness to dwell where you can best feel the breath in your body. Let go of any urge to control, any tendency to manipulate, and simply observe and welcome your breath as it is. Stay in the sensations produced by your breathing: that slight increase in tension when you take in air, that slight release when you expel it. Embrace whatever emotions and thoughts arise as you rest like this.
- At the end of these exercises, invite the participants to gently return to an outward-oriented state of consciousness. This transition is an opportunity to

observe how the autonomic nervous system responds to input from the surroundings and others.

8.4   Setting Homework

The Movements That Suit You

It is now time to introduce the homework assignment for the week. The instructor should provide a handout detailing each of the above poses and their instructions so participants can practice at home. Introduce the homework as follows:

Throughout today's session, we have worked through a series of activities centered on mindful movement. Using the handouts, please review and practice the exercises you completed in class at home as often as possible. Identify the three most meaningful to you. Answer the following questions in writing (see the examples of completed homework in Figure 8.20):

- Which are your favorite asanas?
- How did they affect your nervous system?
- How did you feel after doing them?

Explore asanas with curiosity, fully appreciating their benefits, and make them an integral part of your well-being routine.

GIULIA

Which are my favorite asanas? What impact do they have on my autonomic nervous system?

After the last lesson, I started using movement to get out of sympathetic or dorsal vagal states. I did not use movement before because I didn't know about its regulatory effects. I used breathing and, when possible, cognitive restructuring to calm myself down. However, this did not have much impact, especially when I was in a dorsal vagal state. During the week, something happened that made me go into a sympathetic activation. I was on the subway, there was a big crowd, it was very hot, and in addition, the train doors got stuck. This prevented passengers from leaving the carriages and caused general anxiety. This situation made me very nervous, and I got stressed out. I decided to sit down at that point, and almost immediately, I noticed how stiff my body was—as if I had clammed up. I then placed my hands on my thighs and tried to sit up as straight as possible; I slowly rotated my head to the left and then inhaled. When I exhaled, I rotated my head to the right. By breathing slowly and doing these movements for several minutes, I came out of the sympathetic state. I also noticed that by relaxing my body and keeping an 'open' posture, it was easier to perform cognitive restructuring because I was more lucid, and this allowed me to calm down within a few minutes.

Figure 8.20 Movement: Example of Homework Completed by Participants.

8.5   Closing Ritual and Farewell

The session ends with gratitude to each participant's nervous system and the encouragement to use movement as a regulation resource as often as possible, followed by a collective farewell.

Session 9

A Polyvagal Approach to Life

We have reached the last session before *Safety and Connection Day*, the final stop on the *Wired to Connect* journey. The objective of this session is to encourage participants to build a bridge between the insights gained so far and their everyday lives. They can achieve this by making simple changes to their routine and surroundings – practicing self-massage and selecting food, leisure activities, sleeping habits, and furniture arrangements that promote self-care, steering the autonomic nervous system towards regulation.

The essence of this model is to cultivate a polyvagal approach to life. This endeavor will require constant commitment and attention. It is about creating a new house for yourself, one built on polyvagal foundations that promote psychological, emotional, and physical well-being.

Learning Goals

- Reinforcing the importance of conscious movement as a resource for autonomic regulation through the homework review.
- Understanding how making changes to daily life can foster a polyvagal approach to reality.

Session Framework

1 Session opening and homework review – 60 minutes
2 Polyvagal Module 9 – 60 minutes
3 Homework: Safety and Connection Day preparation – 10 minutes
4 Closing ritual and farewell – 5 minutes

N.B.: As always, the above times are only intended as a guide. The process should be adapted to the group's needs, which we encourage you to prioritize as part of your roadmap.

DOI: 10.4324/9781003560968-14

9.1 Session Opening and Homework Review

After a warm welcome, the instructor gives a brief summary of the previous session and starts the homework review. Invite the group to actively reflect on each other's experiences, enriching their understanding of how conscious movement can represent a resource for nervous system modulation.

9.2 Polyvagal Module 9

In the previous meetings, you led the group through an in-depth exploration of the three golden resources for autonomic regulation: breathing, sound, and movement. But what additional steps can we take to make our lives polyvagal? How can we enhance our co-regulatory potential? What concrete actions can we implement? Today's session aims to provide answers to these questions.

Below, we list a comprehensive range of suggestions, tips, and practical ideas that you can share with participants. Before you pass them on, however, you should try them all out and ponder their effects. From this informed perspective, you will then be better equipped to suggest to the group those options that best align with your sensibilities and the characteristics of the class.

In short, this class will arm participants with a polyvagal toolkit they can rely on after the course.

Tip 1: Eat Well

We are what we eat. Food is an essential component of human life. Our food choices have a decisive impact not only on our health but also on the way we feel. Eating well is another powerful tool for taking care of our autonomic nervous system: it can enhance our mood, alleviate stress, and improve sleep regulation. A healthy diet starts with the ingredients we select, which should ideally be fresh and seasonal. The aim is not to give up food but to learn to balance our intake. Here are some basic tips:

- Vary your food, choosing rice, wheat, potatoes, pulses, meat, fish, and fresh fruit and vegetables.
- Eat wholegrain pasta, rice, and flour.
- Increase your intake of beans and pulses.
- Consume more vegetable soups.
- Opt for juices, smoothies, and fresh fruit extracts with no added sugar.
- Lower your intake of salt and sugar.
- Cut back on alcohol and sweetened drinks.
- Eat less meat, especially red meat.
- Use olive oil rather than butter.

This advice is generally applicable to most individuals. However, if you have specific dietary requirements or concerns, it is advisable to consult a nutritionist for a tailored plan.

Tip 2: Sleep Well

Quality sleep is vital for our health and our psychological well-being. However, many of us feel tired, restless, and unrefreshed when we wake up. Often, this is due to the stress we encounter in our daily lives leading to an over-activation of our autonomic nervous system's protective responses, which can disturb our sleeping patterns. While insomnia is a medical condition that requires proper medical treatment, we can all benefit from improving our sleep hygiene and quality.

Here are ten basic guidelines for achieving restful sleep (Marzano and Montano, 2022, pp. 32–33):

1   *Maintain a regular sleep routine.* Go to bed and get up at the same time every day, within a 20-minute window.
2   *Avoid daytime napping.* Staying awake during the day increases your chances of getting to sleep at night.
3   *If you can't sleep, do not stay in bed for more than ten minutes.* Instead, get up, leave the bedroom, and do something relaxing, like reading a book.
4   *Return to bed only when you feel sleepy.* Do not watch TV in bed. Avoid using electronic devices and ensure all screens are off.
5   *Avoid caffeine and nicotine intake.* The effects of caffeine can last for many hours, causing difficulty drifting off and fragmented sleep. Nicotine is also a stimulant, and it is preferable to avoid smoking in the evening and at night.
6   *Have regular meals before bedtime.* Don't go to bed hungry (hunger can disrupt sleep), and avoid consuming fatty or rich foods in the evening. Opt for lighter evening meals to enhance sleep quality.
7   *Avoid alcohol, especially in the evening.* It may help you fall asleep initially, but it generally increases the chances of nocturnal awakenings and early rising in the morning.
8   *Engage in regular physical activity.* Exercising daily, especially during daylight hours, makes it easier to fall asleep and promotes deep sleep.
9   *Make sure your bedroom is comfortable and quiet.* Your sleep space should be protected and dark enough, with a temperature that is neither too hot nor too cold.
10 *Place your alarm clock out of sight.* Watching the clock when trying to fall asleep or in the middle of the night can be frustrating and cause thoughts and emotions that interfere with sleep.

Tip 3: Get Moving

Many of us lead a sedentary lifestyle. We spend most of our time sitting, often in front of a computer screen. When we commute, it is mostly by car or public transport. When it's finally time for a well-deserved break, we generally end up relaxing on the couch watching a movie. But our bodies are made to move. Regular physical activity not only promotes health but also helps us regulate our autonomic state.

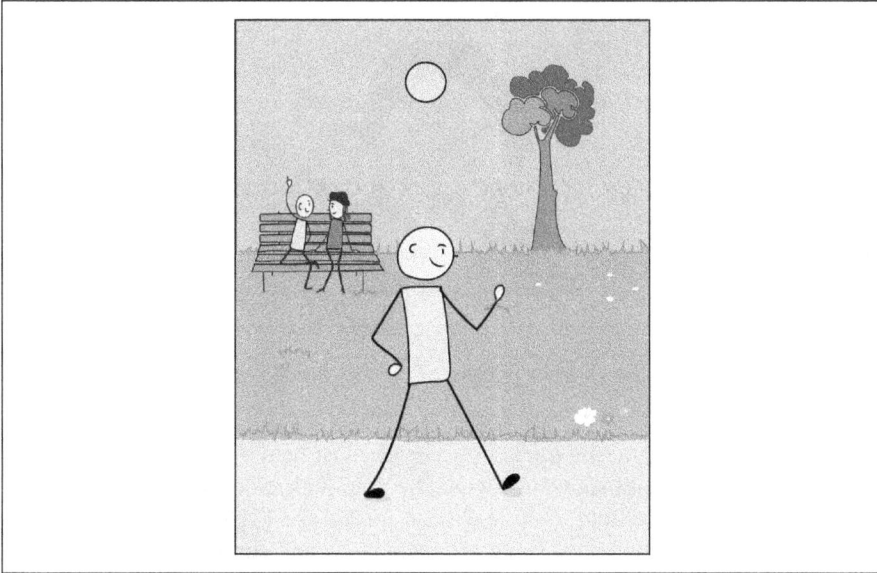

Figure 9.1 The Importance of Movement.

It is not necessary to train like an athlete, but a polyvagal approach to life involves integrating movement into our routine. Choose a type of activity that suits your physical abilities and provides satisfaction (Figure 9.1). The simplest and most affordable solution for everyone is walking. Long brisk walks, alone or – even better – in company, can be extremely beneficial to both your body and your mind.

Tip 4: Give Yourself a Massage

Receiving a massage can be a wonderful and deeply rejuvenating experience for most of us. Contact with another's hands raises awareness of our own body and, consequently, provides an opportunity to really *feel*. As incredible as it may seem, the same sensations can also be experienced through self-massage. Below is a sequence of exercises aimed at stimulating the various sections of the vagus nerve. You've heard of the wonderful effect of acupuncture. Well, now get ready for acupressure: it offers the same benefits but without the needles!

FACE

For this massage, you will mainly use the middle finger of both hands and, to a lesser extent, your index and ring fingers to make circular motions. Your touch should be light and delicate; don't push too hard. Try to apply continuous and comforting pressure (Figure 9.2).

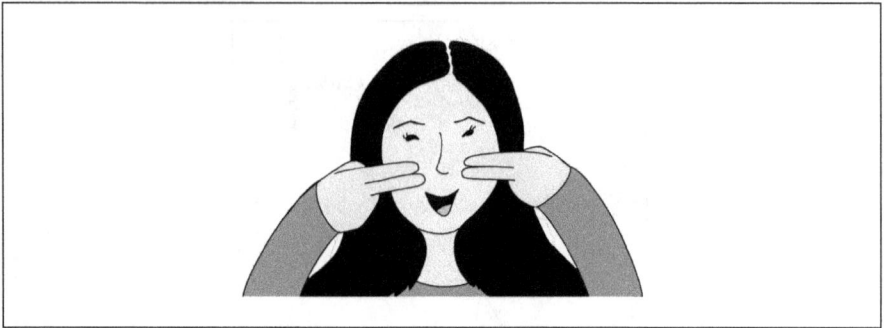

Figure 9.2 Use a Gentle Touch and a Soothing Pressure during Facial Massage.

- Place your fingers at the joints of your jaw, just below your ears. Close your eyes if it helps, and start massaging the area with clockwise rotating movements. We tend to hold a lot of tension in this area. Let your middle fingers gently work out the knots. Breathe consciously, and continue gently for about a minute. Then, reverse the direction of rotation and massage for another minute. As you are doing this, you can also open and close your mouth. Listen to what your body needs and go along with it.
- Place the same fingers below your nostrils, in the space between them and your upper lip. Massage yourself all around your mouth, along your expression lines, in a mustache shape. Once you get to your chin, move back to the base of the nose, continuing with the same motion for about a minute.
- Massage the space between your eyebrows. Choose your dominant hand, left or right. Bring your middle finger and index finger there and gently massage in small circular motions, first in one direction and then in the other. Continue for about a minute. Breathe mindfully, and take note of your experience.
- Using both hands, place your middle fingers on your temples and massage them, using small circular movements in one direction and then the other. Continue for about a minute. As you do, notice your breathing and any sensations that arise.
- Move the same fingers into the hollows inside your ears. Massage in one direction first and then the other. Continue for about a minute. Note the sensations that emerge while you massage yourself like this.

EARS

This form of self-massage is a stretching exercise for the cartilage of the ears.

- Start with your left ear, grasping the top between your left thumb and index finger and the lobe between your right thumb and index finger.
- Pull apart gently for about a minute, breathing consciously and observing your sensations. Repeat the exercise with the other ear.

HEAD

- Using both hands, massage your scalp with the tips of all your fingers as if you are working in shampoo.
- Continue for a couple of minutes, trying to cover the entire surface of your scalp, concentrating on the areas where you feel tension.
- Cover your ears gently with the palms of your hands.
- Use your fingertips to tap the back of your head, moving them upwards and downwards. You should hear a drumming sound.
- Continue for about a minute, breathing consciously and paying attention to all the sensations you feel.

NECK AND SHOULDERS

- Place the fingers of both hands, except the thumbs, at the base of the back of your neck.
- Massage your neck muscles, applying small circular motions with light pressure from your fingertips. Move from the top to the bottom of your neck until you reach the shoulder line.
- Place both hands on your shoulders and massage them, grasping the muscles between your thumbs and fingers and moving from the neck towards the arms.
- Continue with this massage for about a minute, working out the tension. Remember to breathe consciously and pay attention to everything you feel.

CHEST

- Place the palm of your right hand on the left side of your chest, about half a hand's width away from your armpit. Keep your fingers separated and softly resting on your ribs.
- Move just the fingers of your hand up and down, applying light pressure with your middle finger.
- Continue for about a minute, breathing consciously and massaging yourself, paying attention to all your sensations.
- Repeat the exercise on the other side.

ABDOMEN

- Use your dominant hand, left or right. Place it in the center of your belly, over your navel (belly button).

- Massage your abdomen, moving your hand first from left to right, then from top to bottom. Continue for about two minutes and observe all the sensations that arise.
- Using both hands, massage the area around the navel with circular motions, first in one direction and then in the other. Continue in this way, breathing and massaging yourself for about a minute, paying close attention to everything you experience.
- Finish by placing both palms above your navel. Stay in this position for about a minute.

Tip 5: Feel the Cold

A plunge in icy water can have great restorative benefits for your vagus nerve. An alpine lake would be the ideal place for this, but a cold shower can be just as good. Consider ending your daily shower with a blast of cold water or splash some on your face whenever you feel numb or tired. Even running your wrists under the cold tap can be a big help.

Tip 6: Create a Safe Space

Not all environments are created equal. There are some that are noisy, teeming with activity, and therefore overstimulating for our autonomic nervous system, while others inspire serenity, giving our neuroception a reassuring message.

Our homes today are often cramped and shared with other people and/or our pets. Whether large or small, it is essential to rethink our living spaces. The idea is for you to build a home you can love. If a full redesign is impossible, find a corner to transform into a quiet, cozy haven of ventral vagal tranquility. This can become your safe space, a small oasis of calm where you can unwind and regulate your autonomic state.

But what does your safe space need?

- *Order and cleanliness*. Clutter is jarring to the autonomic nervous system. Keeping your safe space clean and tidy will quiet your mind.
- *Color*. Choose your preferred colors, but know that green and blue generally signal safety to our neuroception.
- *Flowers and plants*. There are many benefits to bringing nature indoors. We suggest you create a garden room or corner, concentrating as many plants as possible in the same spot. Place them next to each other and on different levels. Make a display. Choose plants appropriate for your environment and consider using special growth lamps if needed (Figure 9.3).

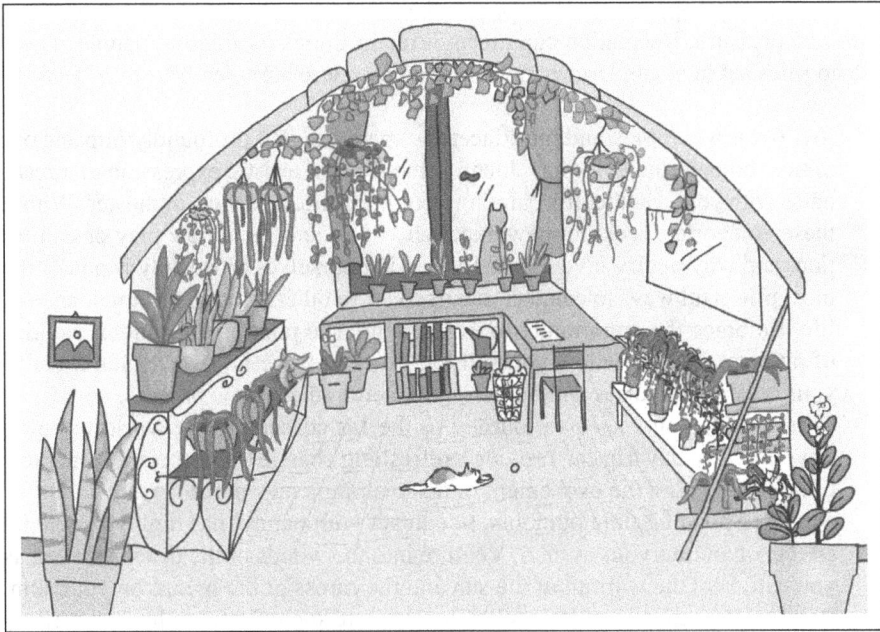

Figure 9.3 Create a Safe Space by Bringing Nature Indoors.

Tip 7: Turn on Play Mode

From an autonomic perspective, entering *play mode* means dwelling in an optimal activation state. That is when the ventral vagal and the sympathetic systems work in sync, the latter under the threshold of fight or flight. (Figure 9.4).

Play is a very broad concept. It can mean different things to different people. You can play an instrument, a game, or a part on stage. Play Mode, however, is mostly a state of mind. It is not so much *what* we are playing that counts, but rather *how*. Regardless of the activities, the focus is on the state we enter as we play: energized, vital, excited, engaged, amazed, joyful, and connected.

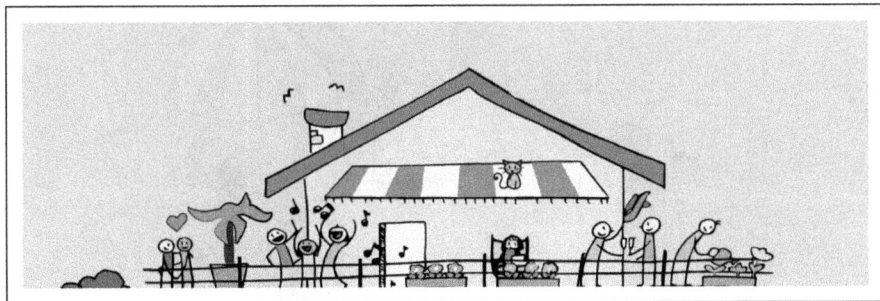

Figure 9.4 Play Mode as an Optimal Activation State.

In a polyvagal approach to life, *play* is the magic word that opens the door to leisure and pleasure. Recreation can mean different things to different people. There are no rules set in stone. Do whatever you enjoy. Here are a few ideas:

- *Art*. Art is a complex and multifaceted experience that profoundly impacts our minds, bodies, and emotions. Identify the form of artistic expression that resonates with you, whether it's painting, sculpture, music, dance, or theater. Within these categories, seek out new experiences: go and see a new play or exhibition, and why not try it yourself? Expressing ourselves artistically is one of the most powerful ways to connect to ourselves, to others, and to the abundance of life. Embrace the opportunity to experiment. The point is to abandon the idea of performance and allow yourself the freedom to be imperfect. Surrender to your creative impulses and immerse yourself in the artistic process.
- *Travel*. You don't need to journey to the far corners of the world to enjoy travel. Even a day trip can provide a refreshing change of perspective, the thrill of adventure, and the excitement of discovering a new place.
- *Nature*. Spending time outdoors, in contact with nature, has highly beneficial effects on our nervous system. Venture into the woods or the beach as often as you can. Feel the warmth of the sun and the caress of the breeze on your skin. Revel in the sensations. If feasible, incorporate some form of physical activity into your outdoor adventures – there's no need for grand plans; even visiting the neighborhood park can be a good start.
- *Water*. We have already noted that cold water is a great resource, but you don't always need to get wet. Look for a stream or body of water – a river, lake, or sea – to visit as often as possible (Figure 9.5). Dive in if you can. Let yourself be rocked by the waves and feel the sensations that pass through you.

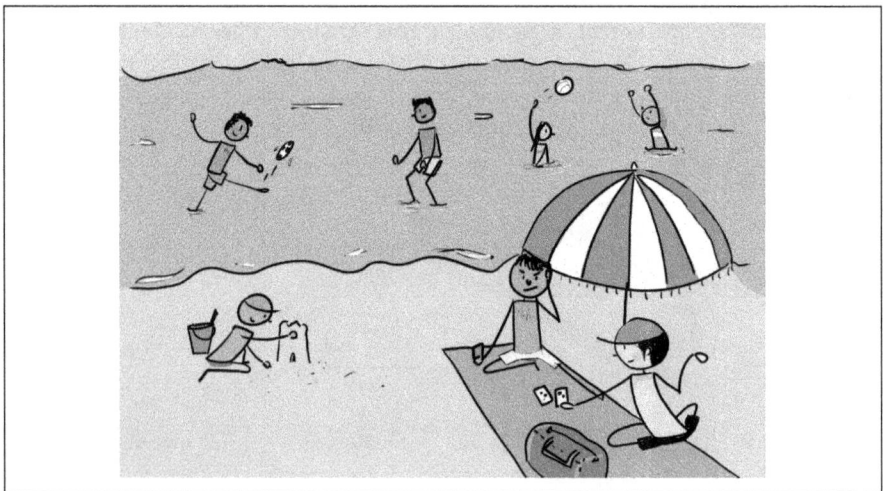

Figure 9.5 Being Close to Water Is Extremely Beneficial for Our Nervous System.

Tip 8: Make Time for Yourself

We have discussed extensively the importance of meaningful relationships for our physical, emotional, and psychological well-being. Yet, for various reasons, we seldom prioritize them. With so many commitments and so little time, our social lives are often the first things to suffer.

Furthermore, even when we are around people, we pay little attention to them, focused as we are on our smartphones. We tend to cultivate virtual friendships at the expense of real ones. We might get lots of "likes" on social media, but we can nevertheless feel detached from others on a deeper level. As we have seen, co-regulation, a biological imperative and a real balm for our nervous system, struggles to be felt through a computer or phone screen. Poor quality relationships, or rather a lack of close bonds, can engender feelings of isolation, negatively impacting our mental health. Relational isolation can send us into a desperate, helpless, frozen dorsal vagal state, like the basement of our Polyvagal House.

That being said, it is crucial to differentiate between loneliness and being alone. Just as we need to make room for love and exchange affection for others, we also need moments to withdraw and reset, with only ourselves for company. Solitude experienced in this way – as a choice or a resource – is *ventral vagal*. It allows us to befriend our inner universe and get in touch with our most authentic desires. It also gives us a foundation of security and connection for creativity. It is an opportunity to grow, reflect, take stock, and look ahead.

Tip 9: Practice Mindfulness

Mindfulness is the art of paying attention to what *is*, lovingly and without judgment. It is a watchful but relaxed look at reality. We live our lives in a hurry. Our sympathetic nervous system drives us to always be doing something, to never stop. Mindfulness is a way to reverse this. It teaches us how to slow down. When we "stop and smell the roses" we begin to notice the pleasant events that illuminate our everyday lives, our *glimmers*. We become aware of and able to bask in beauty in all its various forms. We cultivate a new attitude based on welcoming what *is*, and through it we learn to better face life's adversities.

Moreover, constant attention to breathing – the keystone of mindful meditation – is, in itself, deeply regulating for the nervous system. We are fully aware of ourselves. We experience immobility without falling into the dorsal vagal state. We open ourselves up to a state of connection to ourselves, to others, and to the world around us: a kind of spiritual awakening.

But how do we introduce mindfulness into our life?

- *Reading about it.* Some books can be very useful and inspirational guides to learning how to meditate.
- *Joining a group.* There are many meditation centers offering courses for groups, normally under the guidance of a mindfulness instructor and/or a spiritual teacher.
- *Attending an MBSR course.* The Mindfulness-Based Stress Reduction Program is a structured approach that has scientifically demonstrated benefits. Such courses teach you how to practice mindfulness across eight weeks. There are both online and in-person courses to choose from.

Tip 10: Be Grateful

Mindfulness – the practice of welcoming what is, as it is – is the door to compassion. It is the path that allows us to investigate any of our autonomic nervous system responses with curiosity and the benevolent gaze of an observer.

This is where a new way of being in relationship with ourselves and our autonomic activation patterns begins. We can leave behind self-criticism and the perception of being profoundly wrong. Instead, we can celebrate the intrinsic wisdom of our neuroception and its unique mission: to keep us safe from the very first moment we come into the world.

Cultivating compassion means remembering that our reactions may not be down to us, but rather *what has happened to us.* We must recognize why our bodies and minds were forged in a certain way. Once we stop being judgmental, we make room for gratitude. Despite our troubles, we have lots to be grateful for: first and foremost our nervous system. It watches out for and protects us, allowing us to survive. It gifts us the experience of joy, even amidst the pain, love alongside anger, and safety alongside fear.

When you attune yourself to perceiving the good in the world – the faces of the people you love, the sunlight that warms you, the rain that nourishes the earth, the wind that shakes the leaves, the starry sky above you, and the scent of the flowers below – giving thanks for it daily, you will feel your perception start to shift. The glass, which once seemed half empty, is now invariably full. If you live in gratitude, you are primed for connection and open to the world in all its glory (Figure 9.6). Enjoy it!

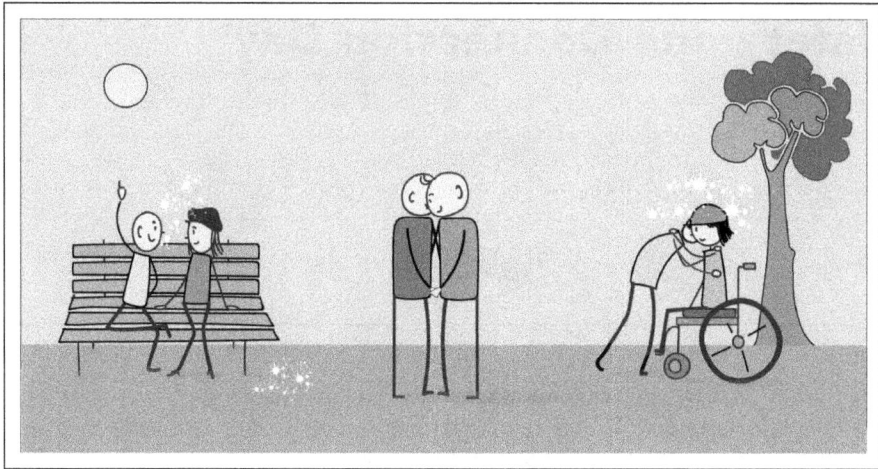

Figure 9.6 Practicing Gratitude Makes Us Feel More Expansive.

9.3   Setting Homework

Preparing for Safety and Connection Day

The program is nearing its end. Hence, the instructor will not assign homework but, instead, prepare the group for the forthcoming intensive class. Encourage attendance in person for *Safety and Connection Day*, even if the course was conducted online. Remind the participants to bring their own lunch, a folder with all the homework they have done, and a pencil case with colored markers. Also, clarify that cell phone use will only be permitted during breaks.

9.4   Closing Ritual and Farewell

For the closing ritual, propose one or two sound, movement, or breathing activities, those most meaningful to the group. As always, express gratitude for each participant's nervous system, encouraging them to integrate these tools into their daily lives. Finish with a collective farewell.

Session 10

Safety and Connection Day

This is the final appointment of *Wired to Connect*. It lasts approximately eight hours and features a wide variety of activities. As mentioned, this session should be attended in person, even if the course was conducted online. Over the previous weeks, participants have learned to modulate their nervous system and actively nurture their biological imperatives for safety and connection. They have built themselves a toolkit that will enable them to reside in ventral vagal energy and deal more effectively with any stressors that they may encounter. Today's meeting serves as both a celebration and an integration of all the techniques learned during the program, providing participants with a comprehensive overview of the positive transformations they have achieved. This is an opportunity for them to fully appreciate and express gratitude for the intrinsic intelligence of their autonomic responses. After all, we have plenty to be thankful for: our newer, more resilient selves, our partners in co-regulation, the earth beneath our feet, and the immense sky above us – a reminder that there is always something greater than ourselves.

The session is also geared towards drawing out one of the most powerful manifestations of connection to the self, a talent that distinguishes us from the other species: our creativity. Participants are encouraged to feel, shape, and honor their biology with playfulness, irony, and beauty by drawing, creating a visual reminder of everything they have learned about their nervous system and themselves.

This is a bittersweet occasion, a watershed marking both an accomplishment and a poignant farewell. Following this session, the group will disband. Therefore, it is essential for the instructor to provide a space for participants to voice any feelings of anxiety or sadness that may naturally emerge. Remind them that a difficult parting is testament to the strength of the co-regulating relationships they have formed with each other. However, they now understand the importance of recruiting other co-regulators among their loved ones, and know how to cultivate and nurture such bonds. They possess the skills to keep on building a supportive polyvagal environment for themselves.

Learning Goals

- Briefly retracing the key content of the course.

DOI: 10.4324/9781003560968-15

- Summarizing the course teachings through visual means.
- Carrying out a range of activities centered on the three golden resources for regulating autonomic states: breathwork, sound, and movement.
- Celebrating the wisdom of our autonomic responses and integrating gratitude as a part of everyday life.

Session Framework

1 Session opening – 15 minutes
2 The activities of the day
   - Building a Polyvagal Village – 60 minutes
   - Guided imagery: thanking your autonomic nervous system – 30 minutes
   - Drawing your autonomic tree – 60 minutes
   - Bee breathing – 10 minutes
   - Your favorite breaths – 60 minutes
   - Mindful movement – 40 minutes
   - Your favorite sounds– 40 minutes
   - Guided imagery: the lotus flower – 30 minutes
   - Saying thank you – 60 minutes
3 Closing ceremony – 5 minutes

10.1   Session Opening

As always, the instructor should prepare the workspace beforehand. Arrange the room with mats and, if desired, cushions or meditation benches. Make sure handouts, paper, markers, and all necessary materials for the various activities are available, and remind participants to bring along all the worksheets they have collected during the course. If you have been conducting the program online, this will be the first opportunity for the group to meet in person. After welcoming them, allow time for introductions and acknowledge the significance of being all together in the same room. Remind them that cell phones should only be used during breaks, if at all. Explain the agenda and schedule of the day.

10.2   The Activities of the Day

A wide variety of activities is proposed to revisit the program from beginning to end, helping participants consolidate the concepts and skills they have learned. Choose the exercises that best suit you and the group, given the time available. Aim to construct a pathway that illustrates the journey undertaken and celebrates where you have arrived together. At the end of each activity, allow time for sharing personal experiences. Again, ask questions that help people reflect on their autonomic world and open up to each other from an underlying state of security and connection.

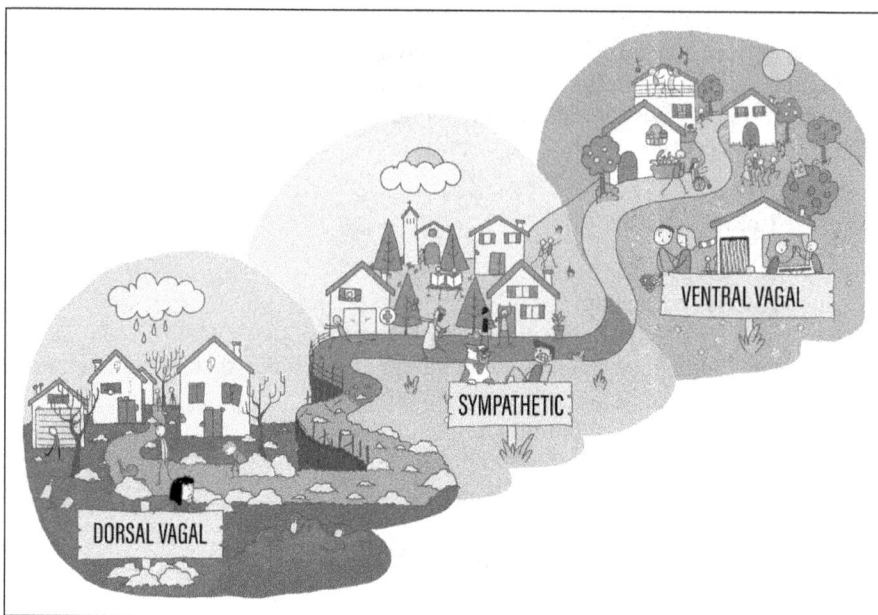

Figure 10.1 The Polyvagal Villages: Another Representation of the Autonomic Landscape.

Activity 1: Building a Polyvagal Village

The first activity involves revisiting the three core principles of Polyvagal Theory – autonomic hierarchy, neuroception, and co-regulation – to consolidate the lessons learned. This can be achieved by introducing a new metaphor: the Polyvagal Villages. While illustrating the theory, create connections to the graphic representations previously used – the Polyvagal House and Autonomic Ladder – and stimulate group discussion. At the end of their polyvagal adventure, participants should be able to take an active role in recalling and expanding upon the various ideas.

Another way to represent our autonomic landscape is to use three villages. As you can see, each village has its unique characteristics, atmosphere, and climate (Figure 10.1). In the dorsal vagal village, it is always raining, the sky is gray, the trees have no leaves, the road is uneven, and the people are sad and lonely, without hope.

Up the winding road, we find the sympathetic village. Here, the weather is unpredictable. The inhabitants are always on high alert, constantly on edge, ready to scream in fear, attack, or run away. Yet, in the upper part of this village, near the path leading to the ventral vagal village, as you can see, residents are engaging in more pleasurable activities. These people are harnessing their sympathetic energy, using it as a resource. They are alert but calm and focused, residing in their optimal activation zone.

The road continues, nicely paved and climbing upwards to the ventral vagal village. Here the sun shines, the trees bear fruit, and the flowerbeds are blooming with vibrancy. The air smells sweet, and life is joyful. People bask in each other's company – hugging, walking, dancing, and supporting each other, experiencing the best that life has to offer.

Distribute a black-and-white outline of the Polyvagal Villages (provided in the online resources) to each participant. Invite them to personalize their drawing using colors, words, or phrases that correspond to their perception of each autonomic state, representing what they have learned about themselves through the course. The road leading from one village to the next can also be decorated to illustrate their triggers (Shadows) and the resources they possess for finding their way back to ventral vagal regulation (Lights) and lingering there. Allow approximately 40 minutes for this activity, monitoring progress and providing support as needed. At the end, participants will be invited to present their personalized version of the three Polyvagal Villages to the group.

Activity 2: Thanking Your Autonomic Nervous System

The day continues with a guided imagery exercise aimed at fostering an attitude of loving kindness towards the intelligence of one's own autonomic nervous system. Invite everyone to sit comfortably but alert – back straight, shoulders relaxed, head raised, and hands softly resting in their lap. Lead them through the exercise using the following prompt:

Allow your eyes to close or your gaze to soften, looking downwards. Try to anchor yourself, observing your breath, noticing the flow of air that goes in and out of your nose. Pay attention to all the sensations in your body. Welcome your next breath by relaxing your abdomen. Breathe in and out with belly soft.

Relax the space between your eyes. Soften the muscles around your mouth, jaw, and tongue. Now, release the tension in your neck and shoulders. Notice what happens to you as you relax.

As you know, breath is your anchor, your lifeline, guiding you back to your ventral vagal home. Ease into just observing your breath for a while, and note how your autonomic nervous system responds while you dwell there.

(Pause for a few seconds)

Try to recall a situation in which you felt slightly scared or threatened, which activated your sympathetic nervous system. This can be something that happened recently or a long time ago. Take care of yourself by ensuring you are selecting one that is not too distressing. Stay there for a while and observe the details: where you were, what you were doing, who you were with. Notice how your sympathetic nervous system stepped in to protect you. Maybe the danger was real, maybe only perceived as such. Feel the sensations inside your body. Try to look at what happened from the position of a compassionate observer. Let your heart open to appreciate the intelligence of the sympathetic branch of your nervous system. You can honor its wisdom by saying:

> I know why you're there. I know why you've taken action. I know your story. I know that even when your activation causes me discomfort, you're just trying to protect me, and I am grateful to you for this.

Repeat these phrases to yourself, make them your own. Speak from the heart, as if you were addressing a loved one. Keep breathing in and out consciously. In and out.

(Pause for two minutes)

Now let this situation fade away into the background, and return to observing your breath for a few cycles. Relax. Observe your breath. In and out. In and out.

Next, remember a time when you felt vulnerable and without resources, when your dorsal vagal system came to your aid. Again, ensure that it isn't a highly distressing episode; it can be recent or long past. Stay there for a while, remember the details. Where were you? What were you doing? Who were you with? Notice how your dorsal vagal system intervened, like a guardian, to safeguard your well-being. Feel the sensations inside. Look at them like a compassionate observer would. Open your heart and express gratitude to this part of your nervous system. Celebrate the intelligence of your dorsal vagal branch by repeating:

> I know why you're there. I know why you've taken action. I know your story. I know that even when your activation causes me discomfort, you're just trying to protect me, and I am grateful to you for this.

Repeat these phrases to yourself, customizing them as you see fit. Say them as if you were addressing a loved one. Remember to breathe consciously. In and out.

(Pause for two minutes)

Now let this situation dissolve away. Return to observing your breathing for a few cycles. Just you and your breath.

Now go up the road to your ventral vagal village. Remember a moment, recent or long ago, when you felt good, connected to yourself, your surroundings, and the people around you. Stay there for a while, observing details about the environment around you. Pay attention to what happens. How does your body respond? What emotions do you feel? What thoughts rise to the surface of your mind? Fully embrace the sensations from within. Open your heart. Express gratitude for the preciousness of your ventral vagal system. Repeat after me:

I know why you're there. I know that I can draw on your energy when I need to. I know that you're my safe haven, where I can thrive and connect. I am grateful to you for this.

Repeat these phrases to yourself, adapting them to suit you. Say them as if you were addressing a loved one. Remember to pay attention to your breath.

(Pause for two minutes)

Bring the activity to a close by inviting participants to open their eyes or lift their gaze. At the end of the experience, allow time for the group to share their comments and feelings.

Activity 3: Drawing Your Autonomic Tree

This exercise is a further opportunity for participants to represent what they have discovered and learned about their autonomic nervous system, this time by drawing a tree (Figure 10.2a shows examples of artworks created by course participants). The previous guided imagery connected them with their autonomic states from the inside. This *embodied perception* of the states themselves will serve as an inspiration for their artistic expression. Lead them into the activity as follows:

In the previous exercise, you once again had the opportunity to build an internal connection to your autonomic nervous system. If that were a tree, how would you draw it? What kind of tree would it be? What would its leaves look like? What kind of trunk would it have? What about its branches? And its roots? Are there any words or short sentences you would like to add to make it even more yours?

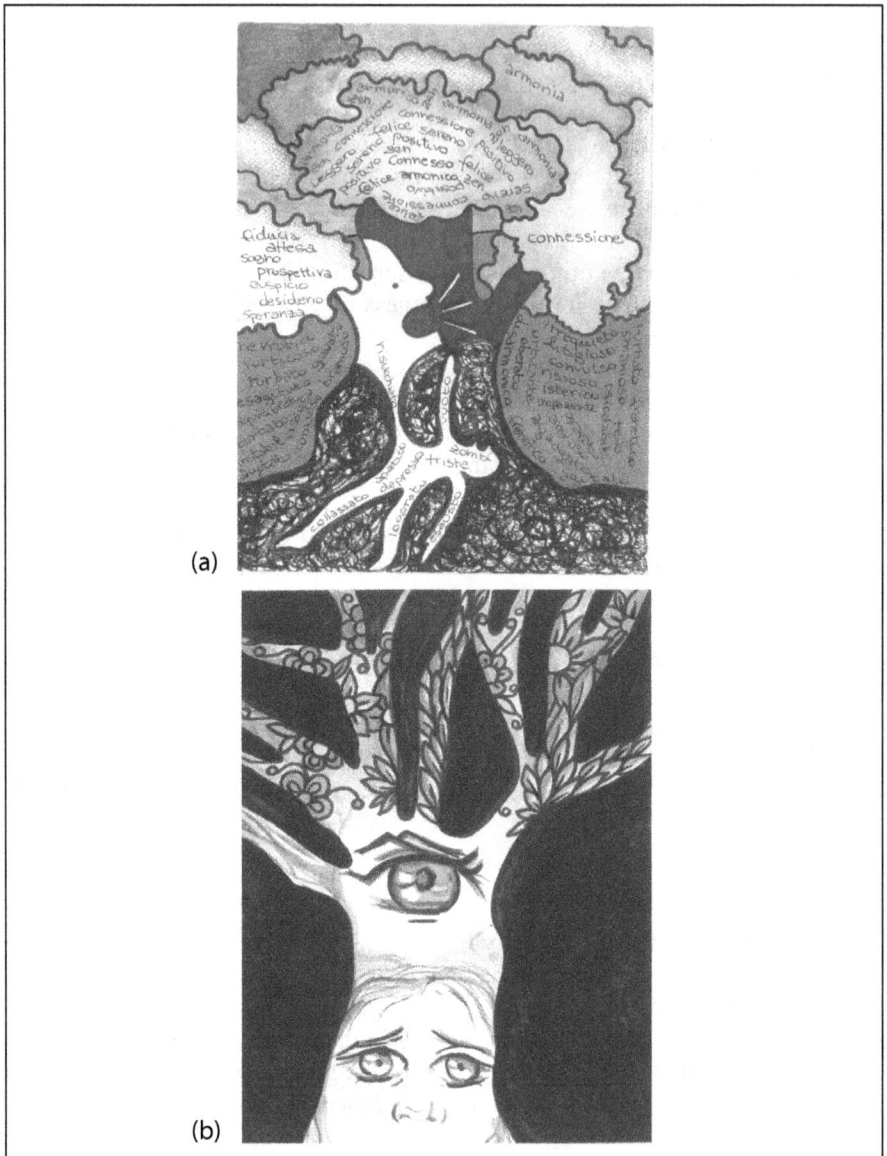

(a)

(b)

Figure 10.2 The Autonomic Tree (a) and (b): Examples of Artworks Created by Course Participants.

Leave the group to work independently for about 30 minutes. Encourage them to unleash their creativity by using different colors, words, and images. Monitor their progress and provide any guidance they may need. Be careful not to influence their output, though: this should be an intensely personal journey.

At the end of the activity, allow each participant to present their Autonomic Tree to the others. Remind them to listen with empathy and to seek benefit from the experiences of others.

Translation

Roots:

Collapsed, Sad, Depressed, Empty, Zombie, Exhausted, Flat

Middle spaces to the sides of the tree:

Spinning, In a Vortex, Shaking, Overwhelmed, Agitated, Nervous, Volatile, Reactive, Resentful, Angry

Upper branches and leaves:

Connection, Trust, Hope, Perspective, Dream, Harmony, Happy, Creative, Zen, Light

---

Activity 4: Bee Breathing

Carried out as a group, this exercise produces a collective sound that is highly moving and soothing for the participants' nervous systems. Such shared experiences have the potential to be extremely co-regulating. This will be especially powerful for online attendees who have not had the opportunity to breathe together as a group before.

Refer to the description in Session 6 for guidance on how to conduct the activity. We recommend practicing Bee Breathing for at least four to five full cycles to fully savor its effects. If participants find the activity enjoyable, feel free to extend it, ensuring that it does not last longer than ten minutes. Afterward, ask if anyone has thoughts or feelings about the experience that they would like to share.

Activity 5: Your Favorite Breaths

For this part of the meeting, select a range of breathing techniques that the participants particularly appreciated. Alternatively, if the group size allows, split participants into smaller groups (three to five people) and allocate them to different parts of the room. Each participant should share with their classmates the breathing technique they found most beneficial, and explain why. The group or subgroup should then practice that technique together for a couple of minutes before moving on to the one selected by the next person. The aim is for everyone to draw inspiration from fellow travelers and experience the power of co-regulation arising from breathing in sync.

Activity 6: Mindful Movement

Next, guide the group through a short mindful movement sequence. The yoga asanas listed below are recommended, but feel free to select others that suit the group's needs from among those described in detail in Session 8:

- Mountain Pose (*tadasana*)
- Standing Crescent Pose (*indudalasana*)
- Standing Forward Bend (*uttanasana*)
- Cat–Cow (*bitilasana marjaryasana*)
- Integration Pose (*shavasana*)

The entire activity should last approximately 40 minutes. To conclude, initiate a group discussion on the impact of these asanas. How did they feel before and after doing them? Have they been able to introduce yoga into their daily lives? If so, how did they do this?

Activity 7: Your Favorite Sounds

The *Safety and Connection Day* continues with a recap of the module dedicated to sound. This segment should last about 40 minutes. As always, select the activities that were most meaningful for the group from those presented in Session 7. We favor Om. This will be a very moving moment, especially for online participants who have not yet meditated together in person. For centuries, the power of this mantra has quieted the minds of monks and regulated the nervous system of all who recite it. When performed together, group members can perceive the vibrations produced by others, opening the door to an experience that can be surprising in many ways. These can be shared as you bring the activity to a close.

Activity 8: The Lotus Flower

As the *Safety and Connection Day* ends, it is the perfect time to lead a guided imagery exploration using the evocative symbol of the lotus flower. Provide the following instructions:

Sit comfortably with your head, neck, and back straight but not stiff. Remember to relax your shoulders. Fold your hands in your lap or, if you prefer, lay them softly on your thighs.

When you feel ready, gently close your eyes and turn your attention to your breath. Let the air in and out of your nose without forcing anything. Allow yourself to breathe naturally as you listen to a story: the story of the lotus flower. As you hear me talking, keep your attention focused within and notice how your autonomic nervous system responds to my words.

(Pause for a few seconds)

The lotus is a wonderful flower that can grow and thrive in the harshest conditions. In many traditions, it symbolizes the capacity for transformation that every living being has. Regardless of our past, our life experiences, or possible adverse situations in the present, we all possess the potential to open up to the beauty of the lotus flower. We can all imagine that we have a lotus seed locked somewhere within us, deeply rooted and ready to blossom.

The lotus seed is shaped like a hard stone, enveloped in a thick shell. It does not sprout in the earth but in water. However, it is not enough to throw one into a puddle or lake to make it grow. You need to crack its surface. This is why the lotus takes root more easily in swamps. The silt and the mud wear away the hard shell, making gaps for new growth to come through. The environment may be harsh, yet the seed does not wither away. It can remain there for weeks, its internal vitality intact. It withstands the elements and stays true to its purpose: to grow and to thrive.

Eventually, the seedling emerges, reaching the sky, transforming waste and sunlight into nourishment and opportunity. Little by little it blooms, growing larger and more majestic. Its petals are fleshy and hardy and provide shelter for frogs and insects, while fish dart playfully among its leaves.

(Pause for a few seconds)

Now, try to envision yourself as a lotus seed. Maybe you are there, still, in murky water, perhaps prey to your nervous system's protective responses. But, like the lotus seed, the time will come for you, too, to turn these experiences to your advantage, emerging from the mud and offering your beauty for the world to see. Nothing can distract you, nothing can stop you.

(Pause for a few seconds)

And so, breath after breath, acknowledge that you, too, have the same potential as the lotus seed. Like the lotus seed, danger or threat can become an opportunity for growth for you. You have the potential to open up and blossom.

Embrace your innate drive for serenity and well-being. Cultivate the determination to rise above the struggles of life, just as the lotus flower does. Draw upon your ventral vagal energy.

(Pause for a few seconds)

Continue to breathe consciously, holding the image of you as a lotus seed close to your heart. When you feel ready, slowly open your eyes.

Wind up the exercise by getting the group to make a lotus flower, or *padma mudra*, with their hands. *Mudras* are symbolic gestures used in yogic practice to complement asanas and guide energy in a specific direction. Lead the participants through the *mudra*, giving the following instructions (Figure 10.3):

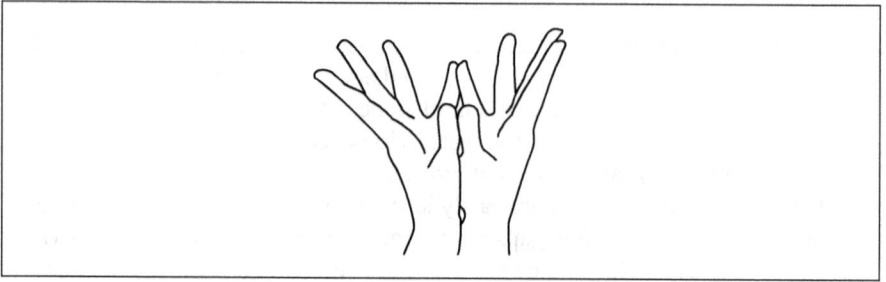

Figure 10.3 Guided Imagery: The Lotus Flower.

- Join your hands together over your heart, placing your palms together.
- Keeping your wrists, thumbs, and little fingers touching each other, open your index fingers, middle fingers, and ring fingers outward, separating them.
- Bring your gaze into your hands and breathe into your blooming lotus flower for four or five full cycles, observing the sensations arising in you.

Unlike the other activities of the day, refrain from asking for feedback and prepare for the next activity, which will build on the energy generated within the group by the guided imagery.

Activity 9: Saying Thank You

As mentioned, expressing gratitude is an important part of a polyvagal life. Give each participant an index card, inviting them to express the following:

- One significant lesson learned on the course
- How *Wired to Connect* has changed them
- Three key takeaways
- A name of a group member they want to thank and why

Encourage them to fill these out anonymously, then mix and distribute the cards randomly. Each participant will read aloud the card they receive.

10.3   Closing Ceremony

We have reached the final closing ritual of the course. We like to finish with the Breath of Joy. Invite the participants to form a circle, holding hands, and guide them through this experience as follows (Figure 10.4):

- Keep holding hands. Raise your arms towards the sky and say together: "Breathe in joy".
- Keep holding hands. Lower your arms and say: "Breathe out joy".

Repeat the sequence three times. At the end, invite participants to let go of each other's hands, paying attention to the impact of this greeting on their autonomic nervous system.

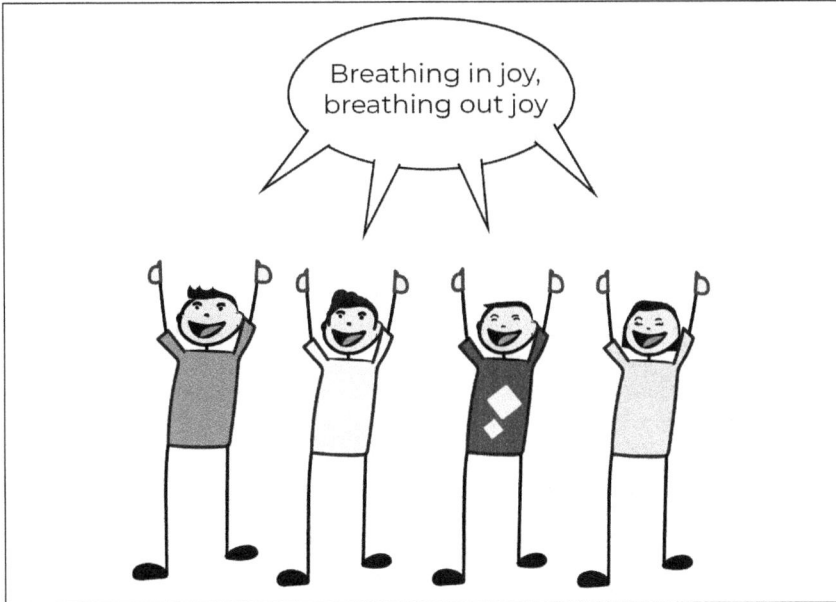

Figure 10.4 Closing Ceremony.

A Final Word

Each of us, by birthright, should start from a position of safety and connection, involving our physical, emotional, and cognitive dimensions. We should be able to open up to and cultivate relationships without fear. We should be capable of fulfilling our ancestral need to meet the gaze, the breath, and, most of all, the heart of others without barriers.

However, many of us have suffered trauma, some more severe or impactful than others. And some of us were hurt by the very people who were supposed to nurture and protect us. Consequently, our nervous systems learned to shy away from contact, leading us to live shielded, isolated lives, cut off from our most vital resource: other human beings. Independence is highly prized by our society, but that doesn't mean that we have to, or indeed should, go it alone. We need human connection, we thrive through bonds of love. Our relationships with others serve as our main source of co-regulation and the most important safety net for our well-being.

Through *Wired to Connect* you have learned to appreciate your autonomic responses, to recognize them as such, and to use them to navigate the path that leads back to the soothing energy of your ventral vagal system. It is here that – like a flower unfurling – you can open up to yourself, others, and reality, and forge those connections that enrich life and make it a joyful journey.

As this course concludes, we hope this book will be a guide and a reference point for you, continuing to speak to you over time. We encourage you to pick it up periodically, to revisit the theory and the exercises, and to work on the relationship you have established with your nervous system, addressing its needs moment by moment. Now you understand that your physiology is not your destiny, and that it is possible to model a new biological foundation for yourself. Show your students or clients how to do the same. Become advocates for this new form of *polyvagal awareness*. You will thus help others to transform discomfort into opportunity and inhabit their skin with heart, body, and mind in the soft embrace of ventral vagal alignment.

DOI: 10.4324/9781003560968-16

Bibliography

Battaglia Damiani, D. (2003). *Anatomia della voce. Tecnica, tradizione, scienza del canto.* Universal Music MGB Publications.

Bennett, B. (2002). *Emotional yoga: How the body can heal the mind.* Fireside.

Boccio, F. J. (2004). *Mindfulness yoga: The awakened union of breath, body, and mind.* Wisdom Publications.

Butera, R., Byron, E., & Elgelid, S. (2015). *Yoga therapy for stress and anxiety.* Llewellyn Publications.

Cella Al-Chamali, G. (2009). *Il grande libro dello yoga: L'equilibrio di corpo e mente attraverso gli insegnamenti dello Yoga Ratna.* Rizzoli.

Cook-Cottone, C. P. (2015). *Mindfulness and yoga for self-regulation: A primer for mental health professionals.* Springer Publishing Company.

Curren, L. A. (2013). *101 trauma-informed interventions: Activities, exercises and assignments to move the client and therapy forward.* Premier Publishing & Media.

Damasio, A. (1994). *Descartes' error: Emotion, reason, and the human brain.* Putnam.

Damasio, A. (1996). The somatic marker hypothesis and the possible functions of the prefrontal cortex. *Philosophical Transactions of the Royal Society of London. Series B: Biological Sciences, 351*(1346), 1413–1420.

Damasio, A. R. (1999). *The feeling of what happens: Body and emotion in the making of consciousness* (1st Harvest). Harcourt.

Damasio, A., & Carvalho, G. B. (2013). The nature of feelings: Evolutionary and neurobiological origins. *Nature reviews neuroscience, 14*(2), 143–152.

Damasio, A. (2021). *Feeling and knowing: Making minds conscious.* Pantheon.

Dana, D. (2018). *The polyvagal theory in therapy: Engaging the rhythm of regulation.* WW Norton & Company.

Dana, D. (2020). *Polyvagal exercises for safety and connection: 50 client-centered practice.* WW Norton & Company.

Dana, D. (2021). *Anchored: How to befriend your nervous system using polyvagal theory.* Sounds True.

Fisher, J. (2019). Sensorimotor psychotherapy in the treatment of trauma. *Practice Innovations, 4*(3), 156.

Geller, S. M. (2018). Therapeutic presence and polyvagal theory: Principles and practices for cultivating effective therapeutic relationships. In S. Porges & D. Dana (Eds.), *Clinical applications of the polyvagal theory: The emergence of polyvagal-informed therapies* (pp. 106–126). W. W. Norton & Company.

Goleman, M., & Moon, C. (2020). *Vagus Nerve. The most comprehensive guide for accessing the natural healing power of your body, activating the healing of vagus nerve, learning self-help exercises for anxiety, trauma and depression.* Independently published.

Hanazawa, H. (2022). Polyvagal theory and its clinical potential. An overview. *Brain Nerve, 74*(8), 1011–1016.

Hartmann, R. (2022). *Daily vagus nerve exercises. Learn how to stimulate and activate the power of the longest nerve in our body, prevent inflammation and calm anxiety with exercises to access your body's natural healing.* Independently published.

Johnson, D. H. (1995). *Bone, breath & gesture: Practices of embodiment.* North Atlantic Books.

Levine, P. A. (2015). *Trauma and memory: Brain and body in a search for the living past: A practical guide for understanding and working with traumatic memory.* North Atlantic Books.

Levine, P. A. (2010). *In an unspoken voice: How the body releases trauma and restores goodness.* North Atlantic Books.

Levine, P.A. (1999). *Healing trauma: Restoring the wisdom of the body.* Audiobook. Sounds True.

Levine, P. A. (1997). *Waking the tiger: Healing trauma—The innate capacity to transform overwhelming experiences.* North Atlantic Books.

Marzano, C., & Montano, A. (2022). *Buonanotte: Esercizi per gestire e superare l'insonnia.* Franco Angeli.

Masunaga, S. (1986). *Zen imagery exercises: Meridian exercises for wholesome living.* Japan Publications, Inc.

McCall, T. (2007). *Yoga as medicine: The yogic prescription for health and healing.* Bantam Books.

Mischke Reeds, M. (2018). *Somatic psychotherapy toolbox: 125 worksheets and exercises to treat trauma & stress.* PESI.

Montano, A. (2022). *Wired to connect. Un approccio polivagale alla vita.* Comunicazione personale nel I Convegno CBT-Italia, Florence.

Montano, A., & Iadeluca, V. (2022). *Meditare con la vita.* Erickson.

Nakamura, T. (1981). *Oriental breathing therapy.* Japan Publications, Inc.

Ogden, P., & Fisher, J. (2015). *Sensorimotor psychotherapy: Interventions for trauma and attachment.* WW Norton & Company.

Owa, I. (2020). *Vagus Nerve* exercises*: A self-help guide to activate the healing power of your Vagus Nerve with* effective *stimulation techniques to relieve anxiety ... depression, chronic illness, inflammations.* Independently published.

Piano, S. (1996). *Enciclopedia dello yoga.* Promolibri Magnanelli.

Porges, S. W. (1985). Spontaneous oscillations in heart rate: Potential index of stress. In S. M. Backs, D. H. Izard, & R. B. Cairns (Eds.), *Animal stress* (pp. 97–111). Springer.

Porges, S. W. (1992). Vagal tone: A physiologic marker of stress vulnerability. *Pediatrics, 90*, 498–504.

Porges, S. W. (1995). Orienting in a defensive world: Mammalian modifications of our evolutionary heritage. *Psychophysiology, 32*, 301–318.

Porges, S. W. (1996). Physiological regulation in high-risk infants: A model for assessment and potential intervention. *Development and Psychopathology, 8*, 43–58.

Porges, S. W. (1998). Love and the evolution of the autonomic nervous system: The polyvagal theory of intimacy. *Psychoneuroendocrinology, 23*, 837–861.

Porges, S. W. (2001). The polyvagal theory: Phylogenetic substrates of a social nervous system. *International Journal of Psychophysiology, 42,* 123–146.

Porges, S. W. (2003). Social engagement and attachment: A phylogenetic perspective. *Annals of the New York Academy of Sciences, 1008,* 31–47.

Porges, S. W. (2004). Neuroception: A subconscious system for detecting threats and safety. *Zero to Three, 24,* 19–24.

Porges, S. W. (2007). The polyvagal perspective. *Biological Psychology, 74,* 116–143.

Porges, S. W. (2009). The polyvagal theory: New insights into adaptive reactions of the autonomic nervous system. *Cleveland Clinical Journal of Medicine, 76,* S86.

Porges, S. W. (2021a). *Polyvagal safety: Attachment, communication, self-regulation.* WW Norton & Company.

Porges, S. W. (2021b). Polyvagal theory: A biobehavioral journey to sociality. *Comprehensive Psychoneuroendocrinology, 7,* 100069.

Porges, S. W., & Dana, D. (2018). *Clinical applications of the polyvagal theory: The emergence of polyvagal-informed therapies.* WW Norton & Company.

Porges, S. W., Bazhenova, O. V., Bal, E., Carlson, N., Sorokin, Y., Heilman, K. J., et al. (2014). Reducing auditory hypersensitivities in autistic spectrum disorder: Preliminary findings evaluating the listening project protocol. *Frontiers in Pediatrics, 2,* 80.

Porges, S. W., Davila, M. I, Lewis, G. F., Kolacz, J., Okonmah-Obazee, S., Hane, A. A., et al. (2019). Autonomic regulation of preterm infants is enhanced by Family Nurture Intervention. *Developmental Psychobiology, 61,* 942–952.

Porges, S. W., Doussard-Roosevelt, J. A., Stifter, C. A., McClenny, B. D., & Riniolo, T. C. (1999). Sleep state and vagal regulation of heart period patterns in the human newborn: An extension of the polyvagal theory. *Psychophysiology, 36,* 14–21.

Porges, S. W., Doussard-Roosevelt, J. A., Portales, A. L., & Greenspan, I. (1996). Infant regulation of the vagal "brake" predicts child behavior problems: A psychobiological model of social behavior. *Developmental Psychobiology, 29,* 697–712.

Porges, S. W., & Furman, S. A. (2011). The early development of the autonomic nervous system provides a neural platform for social behaviour. A polyvagal perspective. *Infant and Child Development, 20,* 106–118.

Porges, S. W., & Lewis, G. F. (2010). The polyvagal hypothesis: Common mechanisms mediating autonomic regulation, vocalizations and listening. *Handbook of Behavioral Neuroscience, 19,* 255–264.

Porges, S. W., & Lipsitt, L. P. (1993). Neonatal responsivity to gustatory stimulation: The gustatory-vagal hypothesis. *Infant Behavior and Development, 16,* 487–494.

Porges, S. W., Macellaio, M., Stanfill, S. D., McCue, K., Lewis, G. F., Harden, E. R., et al. (2013). Respiratory sinus arrhythmia and auditory processing in autism: Modifiable deficits of an integrated social engagement system? *International Journal of Psychophysiology, 88,* 261–270.

Porges, S. W. (2021). *Polyvagal safety: Attachment, communication, self-regulation (IPNB).* WW Norton & Company.

Reed, S. F., Porges, S. W., & Newlin, D. B. (1999). Effect of alcohol on vagal regulation of cardiovascular function: Contributions of the polyvagal theory to the psychophysiology of alcohol. *Experimental and Clinical Psychopharmacology, 7,* 484–492.

Rosenberg. S. (2017). *Accessing the healing power of the vagus nerve: Self-help exercises for anxiety, depression, trauma, and autism.* North Atlantic Books.

Schwartz, A. (2021). *The complex PTSD workbook: A mind-body approach to regaining emotional control and becoming whole.* New Publisher.

Teasdale, J. (2022). *What happens in mindfulness: Inner awakening and embodied cognition.* Guilford Press.

Van der Kolk, B. A. (1996). *The body keeps score: Approaches to the psychobiology of posttraumatic stress disorder.* Penguin Books.

Van der Kolk, B. A. (2003). *Psychological trauma.* American Psychiatric Publishing Inc.

Van Lysebeth, A. (2007) *Pranayama: The Energetics of Breath.* New York: Harmony Publishing.

Van Lysebeth, A. (2012). *Perfeziono lo yoga.* Mursia.

Van Lysebeth, A. (2018). *Imparo lo yoga.* Mursia.

Van Lysebeth, A., & Van Lysebeth, D. (2017). *I miei esercizi di yoga.* Mursia.

Index

Page numbers in *italics* indicate figures

abdominal massage exercise127–28
acupressure 125
art 130
Aum 91, *92*, 142
autonomic activation 50
Autonomic Ladder 11, *12*, 13, 40, *41*,
   45–46, *47–48*, 50, *52–53*, *62–63*, 77,
   103, 136
autonomic nervous system (ANS) xi, xiii,
   5, 7, 8, *10*, 33, *34–35*, 103
   antennas metaphor 42
   dorsal vagal *10*, 11, *12–13*, *41*, 46–47
   house metaphor *35*, 36, 39,
      41–42, 51
   and mixed vagal states 18
   overreacting 59
   and Polyvagal Theory 9
   regulation resources 58–59
   and sound 89
   sympathetic *10*, 11, *12–13*, *41*, 46, 65
   thanking 137–138
   and the vagus nerve 3
   ventral vagal *10*, 11, *12–13*, *41*, 45–46
autonomic responses 36, 64
Autonomic Tree exercise 139, *140*, 141

Beck Depression Inventory (BDI-II) 21
Bee Breathing 80, *83*, *100*, 141
being alone 131
Bhramari 80
body 103, *104*
breath of fire 79–80
breath of joy 77–78, *83*
breathing 71–72, *72–73*, 74, *75–77*, 78, *79*,
   80, *81*, 82–83, 85, 88, 131, 137–138, 141
   see also yoga

breathwork 25, 32, 38, 49, 56, 63, 69–72,
   72–73, 74, *75–77*, 78, *79*, 80, *81*,
   82–83, 85
bridges *54*, 55, 58
bubbles 76

cardiac arrhythmias xi
   "arrhythmic storms" xi
Cat–Cow/Bitilasana–Marjaryasana 115, *115*
central nervous system 7, 8, *34*
change 71, *72*
chanting 91, *92*, 93, *94*, 142
chest massage exercise 127
Child Pose/Balasana *118*
children *37*, 58
   and co-regulation 17
   see also infants
co-regulation 11, *15*, 16, 23, 26–27, 40,
   42–43, *44*, 59, 61, 70, 77–78, *83*, 88, 95,
   96, 123, 131, 134, 136, 141, 145
   and children 17
   and the Social Engagement System 16
Cobra Pose/Bhujangasana *116*
cold water 128, 130
communication, within the *Wired to
   Connect* program 32
compassion 132
conscious movement *see* movement
cooling breath 80, *81*

Dana, Deb xiii, xiv, 4, 12, 16, 19, 40
diaphragm: diaphragmatic breathing 81–82
Difficulties in Emotion Regulation Scale
   (DERS) 21
Downward Dog/Ado Mukha Svanasana
   115, 116

For Product Safety Concerns and Information please contact our EU
representative GPSR@taylorandfrancis.com
Taylor & Francis Verlag GmbH, Kaufingerstraße 24, 80331 München, Germany